HIGH PERFORMANCE LIVING

HIGH PERFORMANCE LIVING

USING THE AOC MODEL TO
IMPROVE EVERY AREA OF LIFE

MIKE HAGERTY

HIGH PERFORMANCE LIVING
Using the AOC Model to Improve Every Area of Life

Copyright © 2025 by Mike Hagerty
All rights reserved. No part of this book may be reproduced, distributed, or transmitted in any form or by any means, including photocopying, recording, or other electronic or mechanical methods, without the written permission from the publisher or author, except as permitted by US copyright law or in the case of brief quotations embodied in a book review.

Disclaimer: This book has been published for the purpose of providing the reader with general information on its subject matter. The author and the publisher believe that the information to be accurate and authoritative at the time of publication. The book is sold with the understanding that neither the author nor the publisher are providing professional advice and the reader should not rely upon this book as such. Every situation is different and professional advice (whether psychological, legal, financial, tax, or otherwise) should only be obtained from a professional licensed in your jurisdiction who has knowledge of the specific facts and circumstances.

Cover Design by Katie Fleming
Interior Layout and Design by Alice Briggs
Editorial Team: Jeffrey Miller, Chloie Benton, Kiska Carr

ISBNs:
Ebook: 979-8-89165-265-1
Paperback: 979-8-89165-266-8
Hardcover: 979-8-89165-267-5

Published by:
Streamline Books
Kansas City, MO
streamlinebookspublishing.com

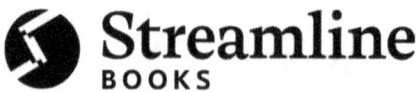

*To everyone striving to reach their highest potential, in honor
of the relentless human spirit that thrives within us all.*

CONTENTS

Author's Note. xi
Introduction. xiii
    The Foundation of Transformation xv
    A Mindset, Not a Checklist. xvii

Part 1: Defining High Performance 1
    Chapter 1: What Is High Performance?. 3
        Focus on Your Game. 4
        Personal and Professional Growth 5
        A Holistic Pursuit 6
    Chapter 2: The Role of Self-Care. 9
        Balancing Work, Recovery, and Growth 10
        From Movement to Mastery 12
        Self-Care as Service 15
    Chapter 3: A Purposeful Self-Care Routine. 17
        Daily Self-Care Habits 18
        Tactics and Tools to Optimize Self-Care 22

Part 2: Awareness 25
Chapter 4: Building Awareness 27
Two Dimensions of Awareness: Data and Reflection ... 28
Awareness in Practice. 30
Mindfulness: The Gateway to Awareness. 32
Awareness Lays the Foundation. 34
Consistent and Continuous Learning 35
Chapter 5: Deepening Awareness 39
Seeing Past Your Blind Spots. 40
Movement and Motivation 42

Part 3: Ownership 45
Chapter 6: Taking Responsibility 47
Four Steps to Owning Your Journey 49
Building a System for Success 52
Chapter 7: Overcoming Barriers to Ownership 55
A Mindset for Action 56
Reflect, Improve, and Stay True. 58

Part 4: Commitment 61
Chapter 8: Prioritizing Action Over Motivation 63
The Power of Blind Faith. 65
Movement Fuels Motivation 67
Resilience + Grit = An Unshakable Foundation. 68
Setting the Tone for the Day 69
Chapter 9: Staying Committed 71
The Role of Goals 72
The Pillars of Goal Setting. 74
Overcoming the Barriers to Commitment. 75
Tracking Progress and Celebrating Wins 77
Tools and Strategies. 78
Tackling Challenges of Any Size 80

CONTENTS

Part 5: Bringing It All Together **83**
    Chapter 10: Integrating AOC into Daily Life 85
        Applying Awareness............................ 86
        Ownership: You Are the Driver.................. 89
        Commitment and the Long Game 92
        Becoming Better So We Can Give More 98
    Chapter 11: Sustaining High Performance 99
        Self-Care Is Nonnegotiable 100
        Just Start Somewhere.......................... 101
        The Power of Showing Up...................... 102

Conclusion..103

Resources...105
    Fifty Habits and Behaviors of High Performers 105
    Awareness, Ownership, Commitment (AOC) Model
    Assessment Tool 109

Recommended Reading List 113

Acknowledgments 117

About the Author......................................119

AUTHOR'S NOTE

BEFORE YOU TURN the page to Chapter One, I encourage you to pause and complete the AOC (Awareness, Ownership, Commitment) self-assessment. This isn't just a warm-up exercise—it's your first step toward High Performance. The assessment is designed to give you a clear picture of where you currently stand in each of the three core areas. It's not about passing or failing. It's about getting honest with yourself—because true growth starts with awareness.

In fact, completing this inventory is an act of Awareness in itself. It asks you to slow down, reflect, and take an honest look at the habits, mindset, and patterns that may be helping—or hindering—your progress. High Performance doesn't happen by accident. It begins when we acknowledge where we are, so we can build a path toward where we want to go.

You'll find the AOC assessment toward the end of this book, where it's easy to revisit later. I encourage you to take it now as your starting point—and again after you've finished the chapters—to measure how far you've come. Give it the time it deserves, and let it ground you in the mindset needed to get the most out of what comes next.

INTRODUCTION

HIGH PERFORMANCE MAY feel like it's out of reach, something that is reserved for the elite few. It's the realm of superstar athletes shattering records, CEOs revolutionizing industries, or artists creating masterpieces. It's easy to assume high performers are different from the rest of us, blessed with rare talent or some secret ingredient we just don't have. But the truth is high performance isn't exclusive to any select group. It's not about being lucky or gifted, and it doesn't require you to be born into greatness.

After years of coaching athletes and working with people from all walks of life, I've learned that high performance isn't a mysterious quality. It's a process. A formula. And the best part is that it's a formula that *anyone* can follow. That means you, too, can unlock extraordinary results, no matter where you're starting from. No, high performance isn't reserved for the chosen few—it's a choice you can make today.

This is where the **AOC model** comes in. AOC stands for **awareness, ownership, and commitment**. Picture a Venn diagram with these three elements overlapping. In the center where they overlap, that's where you find high performance. Whether you're managing a team, running a household, or pursuing athletic goals, this model can help you unlock your greatest potential.

Here's how it works.

It all starts with **awareness**. You can't fix what you don't fully understand. Building awareness relies on two key elements: hard data and instinct. Data provides your baseline. In fitness, this might be your cholesterol levels or body composition. In business, it's your KPIs or revenue figures. These numbers offer an honest snapshot of where you stand, and the numbers don't lie.

But data alone can't give you the full picture. You also need to trust your instincts. What does your gut tell you when something feels off? Perhaps you're constantly fatigued, or you sense your career is stalling. True awareness comes from combining these forces, using both data and intuition to create a clear understanding of what's working and what needs to change.

From awareness, we move to **ownership**. This is where many people falter. It's easy to blame external factors when things don't go well—your boss, your coworkers, your family, your circumstances, society as a whole. But ownership is about taking responsibility for your outcomes. If your performance is lacking, ask yourself, *What can I do to change this?* High performers don't make excuses—they take action. For an athlete, that might mean finding better training partners. For a professional, it could be seeking feedback or additional resources. However, ownership is also about looking inward and realizing that the power to improve lies within you.

Finally, there's **commitment**, the glue that holds it all together. Commitment is where the rubber meets the road. It's not enough to dabble in your goals. You need to go all in on the things that matter most to you. Whether it's your health, relationships, or career, commitment requires consistent focus and effort. On a scale of one to ten, your commitment needs to be a nine or ten to drive meaningful

INTRODUCTION

change. High performers know that true growth happens when you invest deeply and stay the course.

At the foundation of all this lies **self-care**. You can't perform at your best if you're running on fumes. Just like a car requires fuel and maintenance, you need to invest in your overall well-being to stay functional and strong. This means focusing on the basics like getting enough sleep, eating well, and staying active while also incorporating practices that nurture your mental and emotional health, such as meditation or simply carving out moments of quiet for yourself. Self-care isn't a luxury—it's a necessity. Without it, the entire AOC model begins to unravel.

High performance isn't a mystery or a matter of luck. It's a deliberate process, and the AOC model of awareness, ownership, and commitment lays out the path. Built on a foundation of self-care, this approach unlocks potential you may not even realize you have. You see, high performance isn't about being extraordinary or lucky. It's about making the choice to show up, take responsibility, and commit to what matters most. So, what's holding you back from getting started?

THE FOUNDATION OF TRANSFORMATION

In 1983, I took over the wrestling program at the University of Central Missouri, a program that was on the brink of extinction. The athletic director had nearly shut it down, and with just one scholarship and a roster of forty wrestlers, morale was abysmally low. My first task was to bring *awareness* by taking a brutally honest look at the program's poor condition. We were underfunded and overlooked, struggling to operate with lukewarm commitment from athletes who were mostly juggling part-time jobs. But awareness also meant spotting opportunities. I realized we could lean into our underdog status and embrace it as a motivator to disrupt those low expectations.

With awareness in place, I had to embrace *ownership*. No one was coming to save this program. It wasn't the athletic director's problem or the athletes' fault. It was my responsibility. Ownership meant finding creative solutions, like hosting events to attract attention, recruiting strategically with limited scholarships, and putting in countless hours to train and inspire the team. By taking full responsibility and then *committing* to a course of action, I began to reshape the program's future.

This pattern repeated in 1989 when I became manager of coaches' education at USA Wrestling in Colorado Springs. The program was in disarray. Records were missing, and systems were outdated. They had no clear direction. Again, *awareness* was the starting point. I analyzed hard data to understand participation trends and relied on my instincts to identify a need for a bold pivot. We partnered with a national coaching education program, combining our efforts to craft a cohesive and powerful strategy. Taking ownership of this transformation meant fostering stronger relationships and strategically coordinating resources while, at the same time, overcoming the natural resistance to change. The outcome was a rejuvenated program that achieved nationwide reach.

Commitment is where transformation takes root, and it has played a critical role throughout my career. When I returned to the Midwest in 1993 to coach at Blue Springs High School, I inherited a program with potential but lacking momentum. After assessing the situation (*awareness*) and taking responsibility for the program's future (*ownership*), it was time to make a *commitment*.

We overhauled the youth program despite resistance from the community and set a bold five-year goal to win a state championship. While it wasn't an overnight success, we worked tirelessly. Late nights, detailed recruiting strategies, and an unwavering belief in our vision eventually paid off. By year five, we were runners-up, and in year six, we claimed the title.

INTRODUCTION

Most recently, I have moved into health and high performance coaching, but the *commitment* pillar continues to guide my approach. Whether I'm helping individuals define their goals or supporting groups through significant change, I always emphasize the importance of creating sustainable systems and cultivating habits that drive progress. High performance demands dedication and persistence. It's not about striving for perfection but about showing up with intention and putting in the work day after day.

The AOC model isn't just a framework; it's a way of life. Whether you're an athlete, a business leader, or someone striving for personal growth, these principles can guide you to extraordinary results. I've lived it, tested it, and refined it. Now it's your turn to make it your own.

A Mindset, Not a Checklist

High performance isn't about checking off a list of tasks or following a rigid formula. It's not as simple as doing A, B, and C and expecting transformative results. While the AOC model provides some powerful, actionable steps you can take, it's important to remember that true high performance comes from adopting a mindset that is open to opportunities and embraces growth and resilience. It's ultimately about how you approach each day and how you think about challenges.

At its core, high performance starts with what you expect of yourself. Do you believe that change is possible? Do you own your current circumstances, both the wins and the losses? Do you believe that if you become truly aware of your strengths, weaknesses, and opportunities, you can take meaningful action? These are not one-time questions. They need to become daily reflections. You need to embrace the idea that growth is always possible, that setbacks are learning opportunities, and that progress is within reach, no matter where you are currently.

This belief is closely tied to Carol Dweck's concept of a *growth mindset,* a perspective that sees potential and embraces change. With a growth mindset, you understand that even if you haven't been fully aware of your circumstances before, you can cultivate awareness now. If you haven't owned your challenges in the past, you can start today. And if your commitment has wavered, you can strengthen it by taking small, intentional steps forward.

On the flip side, a *fixed mindset*—the belief that your abilities, circumstances, or outcomes are static—can be a major roadblock. Statements like, "That's just not for me," or, "I've tried before, and it didn't work," reflect a mindset that limits potential. These negative tones can overshadow even the best plans and techniques. As a coach, one of my most important tasks is helping people shift from a fixed mindset to a growth mindset. Without that shift, real, lasting change is highly unlikely.[2]

High performance isn't just about what you do. It's about how you think. When you believe in the possibility of growth, take ownership of your path, and commit to consistent effort, you unlock your potential to achieve extraordinary results. Again, this isn't reserved for the elite. High performance is available to anyone willing to adopt the mindset of a high performer—including you.

---

2   Carol S. Dweck, *Mindset: The New Psychology of Success* (New York: Random House, 2006).

HIGH PERFORMANCE LIVING

Part One

DEFINING HIGH PERFORMANCE

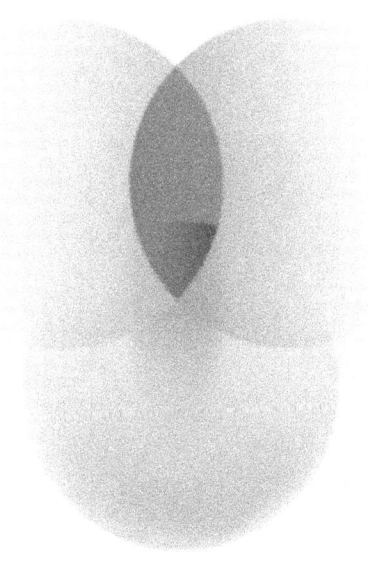

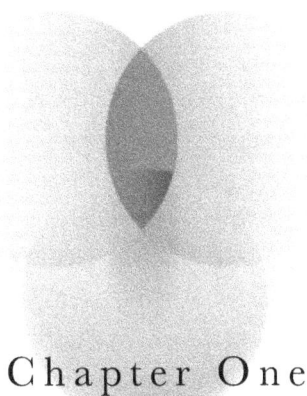

Chapter One

WHAT IS HIGH PERFORMANCE?

THINK ABOUT THE kinds of people we admire from afar. They tend to be visionary leaders, elite athletes, or maybe groundbreaking creatives who produce amazing works of art. People like that sometimes feel superhuman. They achieve things that most of us can only dream about, and we generally assume that they possess some innate abilities or secret ingredients that we do not. But the reality is high performance isn't the result of innate talent or blind luck. Anyone who combines the right mindset with good habits and dedication can achieve far more than they ever thought possible.

Take wrestling, for example, a sport where raw talent alone rarely leads to success. In wrestling, the most successful athletes aren't always the most naturally gifted. They're the ones who engage in disciplined habits and stay consistent. They become brutally aware of their current abilities, but they own the responsibility of improvement and commit to daily effort. The same is true outside the wrestling mat. Whether you're a teacher, a parent, or a business professional, success follows a similar formula.

So high performance isn't about perfection or natural brilliance. It's about building a process that works. If your goal is to get in shape, don't start with an unrealistic workout plan. For the first two weeks, simply put on your workout shoes each day. By week three, pack your gym bag. By week four, go to the gym. Small, manageable steps create sustainable habits. High performance doesn't require a dramatic leap but consistent action.

Focus on Your Game

One of the greatest obstacles to high performance is *comparison*. It's tempting to look at others and think, *I'll never be as good as them.* Look, you don't have to be the best in the world to achieve great things. You just need to strive to become the best in *your* world. Comparing yourself to others dilutes your energy and focus, so instead, prioritize your own unique journey.

Having mentors and role models is helpful, of course, but remember: Their path isn't your path. The strategies and systems that work for someone else may not be what you need. So you need to understand your own goals, challenges, and opportunities. When you stop measuring yourself against others and focus on your own game, you set yourself up for meaningful personal success.

Anyone willing to adopt the right mindset and take intentional steps can achieve great things. High performers aren't extraordinary people—they're ordinary people who do ordinary things extraordinarily well. With awareness, ownership, and commitment, you can tap into your potential and excel in your own world. Yes, high performance is accessible to you, no matter where you're starting from.

Personal and Professional Growth

It's a common misconception that personal growth and professional growth are entirely separate pursuits. We often hear people talk about "personal development" and "professional development" as if they belong to two different worlds. But in reality, the two are deeply intertwined, feeding into and reinforcing each other in powerful ways. When one area thrives, it often boosts the other. Conversely, when one struggles, it tends to pull the other down with it.

If you're not working to become the best version of yourself personally, how can you truly excel professionally? Sure, you might achieve short-term wins by relying on innate skills or past experience, but over time, this approach runs out of steam. Energy and motivation inevitably wane, which can lead to procrastination and a creeping sense of apathy. Projects stall, goals lose their urgency, and that sense of fulfillment you crave becomes harder to find.

Sustained energy is at the core of sustained success. When you prioritize self-care and personal growth, you build the resilience and vitality you need to excel in your professional role as well.

The same principles hold true for organizations. Just as individuals benefit from awareness, ownership, and commitment, so do businesses. A company that takes the time to understand its current state, own its strengths and weaknesses, and commit to deliberate improvement can achieve extraordinary results. When leaders invest not just in profits but in culture, values, and well-being, they create a ripple effect that energizes teams and drives innovation.

Ultimately, personal and professional growth are two sides of the same coin. Investing in yourself personally pays dividends professionally, and when professional success aligns with personal well-being, the synergy can be transformative. This is about more than just achieving goals. It's about creating lives and careers that feel deeply fulfilling and purpose-driven. When you thrive personally, you show up stronger, more creative, and more focused, and that momentum carries into everything you do.

A Holistic Pursuit

Achieving high performance doesn't require hiring expensive trainers, buying magic supplements, or using secret hacks. You just need to adopt a holistic approach that taps into the simple, often overlooked elements of a healthy, balanced life.

In my work with clients, I emphasize starting with a few of the most basic things: *breath, water, movement,* and *nutrition*. These foundational elements are accessible to everyone and can have a deep impact when approached mindfully.

- **Breath:** Harnessing breathwork can reduce stress, improve focus, and enhance overall well-being. Something as simple as mindful breathing for a few minutes each day can reset your body and mind. I emphasize two basic techniques, box breathing and 4/7/8. Box breathing is performed by a four-second inhalation, four-second hold, four-second exhalation, four-second hold, repeat. The 4/7/8 is performed with four-second inhalation, seven-second hold, eight-second exhalation, repeat. Repeating eight to ten cycles will do wonders in helping you reach a more parasympathetic state.
- **Movement:** You don't need a fancy gym membership to incorporate movement into your day. Walk up and down stairs, take a stroll outside, or do some light stretching. Consistent, intentional movement is more effective than sporadic, high-intensity bursts.
- **Water:** Staying hydrated might sound basic, but it's a major priority related to both physical and mental high performance. Drink good, clean water throughout the day to keep your body and brain functioning at their best.

- **Nutrition:** Eat as close to nature as possible. Whether you follow a specific dietary approach like keto, paleo, or vegetarianism, the focus should always be on whole, minimally processed foods.

A holistic approach doesn't mean you need to overhaul your life overnight. Again, you can ease into it. Focus on building one habit at a time. For example, begin with something as simple as drinking an extra glass of water each day or taking a ten-minute walk after meals. These small, consistent actions compound into significant results over time.

One of the biggest traps I see people fall into is searching for a magic bullet, maybe a single supplement or diet that will solve all of their problems. The reality is high performance is about embracing simplicity and consistency. It's about doing the basics well and doing them often. When you pair the AOC model with a holistic approach to well-being, you unlock the potential to thrive in every area of your life.

Remember: Success isn't reserved for a select few. It's accessible to anyone willing to do the work, focus on the fundamentals, and commit to the journey. Start today. Select one healthy habit and incorporate it into your life. That single step is going to help you build momentum toward more substantial changes down the road.

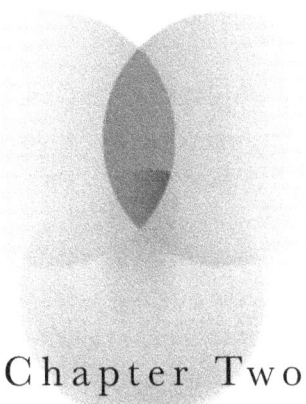

Chapter Two

THE ROLE OF SELF-CARE

WHEN I FIRST set out to write this book, my original focus was primarily on self-care. It was the central theme, the premises of what I wanted to share. Over time, as my ideas evolved into what I now call the AOC model, self-care remained the bedrock upon which everything else is built. Why? Because self-care is the foundation of high performance, and without it, achieving sustained excellence in any area of life becomes incredibly difficult, if not impossible.

Consider the lives of high performers in any field. Read their biographies and study their habits, and you'll find that almost all of them prioritize some form of self-care. Whether it's physical, mental, or emotional, self-care is an essential mindset that grows and adapts with high performers over time. However, self-care isn't often taught. You won't find a "Self-Care 101" class in most schools or universities unless you're in a highly specialized program. For many of us, the journey toward self-care begins through innate curiosity or the hard lessons of experience. But the good news is it's a process you can start with small, manageable steps.

Take, for example, *movement*, one of the core components of self-care. If you want to take care of yourself, you have to start moving. For some, this begins as simply as putting on their sneakers and walking around the block. Over time, that seemingly minor action can grow into a full-fledged exercise routine that transforms both body and mind.

You have to start somewhere. One of my favorite examples comes from a program, WrestlingMS www.wrestlingms.org I've been involved with for over a decade. We help individuals with with multiple sclerosis (MS) regain mobility by getting them on bicycles. Often, their first ride may be less than a mile ride on the trail. But as they develop over time, these same individuals are eventually riding hundreds of miles each week. The progression is nothing short of inspiring and proves that small, intentional steps can lead to remarkable growth.

BALANCING WORK, RECOVERY, AND GROWTH

To be clear, when I talk about self-care, I'm talking about embracing the whole package, including exercise, movement, recovery practices like massage and meditation, and even breathwork. The goal is to achieve a balance between pushing your limits and allowing yourself the necessary time to recharge. Scientifically, this boils down to balancing your *sympathetic* (fight-or-flight) nervous system and *parasympathetic* (rest-and-recover) nervous system. If you overwork without proper recovery, you risk burnout. If you underwork, growth stalls. High performers master this delicate balance, which is why self-care is a nonnegotiable part of their lives.

THE ROLE OF SELF-CARE

Of course, if you're going to master this balance, you need to understand the power of nutrition. Nutrition deserves a chapter of its own within the realm of self-care. Food is more than sustenance—it's fuel for the body, mind, and spirit. High-quality nutrition gives you mental clarity and contributes to your emotional well-being. Without it, achieving high performance in any aspect of life becomes an uphill battle.

Yet, nutrition is often misunderstood. Some athletes believe they can "burn off" poor food choices, but this is a misconception. The quality of what you put into your body matters deeply. Think of your body as a high performance car. Would you put low-grade fuel in a Ferrari? Of course not. Similarly, our bodies demand high-grade nourishment to perform at their best.

Protein, for example, becomes increasingly important as we age, yet many people consume less of it when they need more. Studies in sports nutrition suggest that consuming up to 0.8–1.0 grams of protein per pound of body weight can help maintain muscle mass, support recovery, and boost overall health.[2] So you really need to evaluate whether your nutrition is serving your goals and adjust accordingly.

A common pitfall I see is the "cheat-day" mentality. Popular advice often advocates an 80/20 approach of being disciplined most of the time while leaving room for indulgence, but this can backfire. Cheat days all too often become permission slips for consuming highly toxic foods that derail your progress. As a result, instead of setting yourself up for success on Monday, you're left undoing the damage from the weekend.

Rather than a cheat day, I recommend adopting a daily, mindful approach. Ask yourself, *Is this food serving me?* If the answer is yes, then you're fueling your journey to high performance. If not, make a conscious decision about whether or not to consume it, understanding

---

[2] Michigan State University Extension, "Protein Intake for Athletes," accessed January 7, 2025, https://www.canr.msu.edu/news/protein_intake_for_athletes.

the trade-offs. An approach like this builds *awareness*, one of the three pillars of the AOC model.

As with anything, instead of trying to make sudden, radical changes to your life, I always encourage people to begin taking small steps. That includes nutrition. Whether you're an athlete, a CEO, or simply someone striving to be better, begin with one thing, stay consistent, and always ask yourself, *Is this serving my growth?*

So when it comes to self-care, what's your first step going to be? Maybe it's finally scheduling that check-up you've been putting off. Maybe it's swapping out processed snacks for whole foods. Or perhaps it's finally scheduling that massage you've been putting off. Wherever you begin, remember that self-care is not a destination—it's a lifelong journey, and every step forward counts.

With that in mind, let's look deeper at a few specific areas where you can begin taking incremental movement toward high performance. We'll start with *movement*.

FROM MOVEMENT TO MASTERY

When most people decide to level up their lives and become high performers, the first thing that comes to mind is exercise. While that's a noble goal, diving headfirst into an intense workout regimen can be like trying to take a car from zero to one hundred miles per hour in an instant. It's a recipe for burnout—or worse, injury. That's why I believe the real magic lies in starting small. Remember: *Movement* is the key!

Movement is the foundation of fitness, and it's accessible to everyone. You don't have to run out and join a gym or sign up for a marathon. Just start taking steps—literally. Park farther away from the store. Take the stairs instead of the escalator. Step outside and feel the sun on your face for a moment. These small choices add up over time and create a powerful habit of incorporating more activity into your day.

THE ROLE OF SELF-CARE

Personally, I'm a huge advocate for walking. Not only is it easy on the joints, but it also serves as a perfect way of combining activities. Whether I'm listening to podcasts, brainstorming ideas, or simply enjoying the outdoors, walking allows me to move my body while engaging my mind. It's a low-intensity activity that anyone can do, yet its benefits are significant.

Emerging science supports the idea that low-intensity activities like walking are better for overall health than long sessions of sustained cardio.[3] High-intensity cardio, while beneficial in moderation, can be *catabolic*, meaning it breaks down muscle tissue over time. This isn't necessarily bad occasionally, but consistently engaging in high-intensity cardio without balancing it with recovery can lead to muscle loss.

On the other hand, activities like walking, light cycling, and zone 2 training (exercises performed at a conversational pace) promote longevity and preserve muscle mass. This is especially important as we age because muscle plays a critical role in glucose metabolism, stability, and preventing conditions like insulin resistance and diabetes.

Once you've built a habit of movement into your routine, you can level up with *strength training*. Strength exercises help maintain muscle mass and improve stability while also promoting long-term health. Start small, maybe two days a week, and focus on what you enjoy, whether that's resistance bands, free weights, or bodyweight exercises. Just be consistent.

As you progress, increase to four or five days of strength training per week. Combine this with your baseline movement (e.g., walking, light cycling), and you're setting yourself up for success. Dr. Peter Attia, a leading voice in longevity, emphasizes that strength training

---

[3] Verywell Health, "Is It Time to Ditch HIIT for Steady-State Cardio?" accessed January 7, 2025, https://www.verywellhealth.com/hiit-workout-vs-steady-state-cardio-8760240

combined with VO2 max training (a measure of your cardiovascular fitness) is the ultimate formula for staving off chronic illnesses like heart disease and cognitive decline.[4]

High-intensity interval training (HIIT) is where things get really exciting. These workouts, which involve short bursts of intense effort followed by brief recovery periods, are incredibly efficient. They're quick, effective, and can be adapted to nearly any form of exercise, from sprinting and cycling to burpees and jump rope.

For example, a classic HIIT format might involve twenty seconds of all-out effort followed by ten seconds of active rest, repeated for fifteen to twenty minutes. This approach, often called "Tabata training", can deliver exceptional results in a fraction of the time required for traditional cardio. Plus, it's adaptable. Whether you're a beginner or an experienced athlete, you can tailor HIIT to match your fitness level.

A BALANCED FITNESS PLAN FOR HIGH PERFORMANCE

Here's a sample fitness plan to strive toward:

1. **Baseline Movement (Zone 2 Training):**
   - Five to six days per week, thirty minutes per session.
   - Examples: Walking, light cycling, or casual swimming.
2. **Strength Training:**
   - Four to five days per week, twenty to thirty minutes per session.
   - Focus on compound movements, resistance bands, or body-weight exercises.
3. **High-Intensity Workouts (HIIT):**

---

[4] George Parker, "Why VO$_2$ Max and Strength Training Are Key to Longevity and Health ," Peregrune, accessed January 7, 2025, https://www.peregrune.com/blogs/peregruneblog/b-why-vo2-max-and-strength-training-are-key-to-longevity-and-health-b.

- One to two days per week, fifteen to twenty minutes per session.
- Examples: Sprints, burpees, or interval cycling.

This balanced approach ensures you're covering all the bases—building muscle, improving cardiovascular health, and maintaining mobility—while avoiding overtraining.

Investing in movement and exercise isn't just about improving your physical health. The mental and emotional benefits are equally significant. Regular movement releases endorphins and reduces stress. This makes it a form of self-care that spills over into every aspect of your life, making you more energized, focused, and resilient. And the best part is, you don't have to start big. Like I said, start with a single walk. Add a few push-ups. Take the stairs. These small steps create momentum, and before you know it, you'll have built a fitness routine that not only fits your life but enhances it.

Remember: The journey to high performance begins with movement. So lace up your shoes and take that first step.

Self-Care as Service

When most people think about self-care, they imagine it as a purely personal journey—something that's solely about improving their own health, happiness, and performance. And while it does improve those areas of your personal life, there's another layer to self-care: *being a role model*. Whether you're leading a team, guiding your family, or simply trying to set a positive example for those around you, how you care for yourself impacts more than just your own life.

For many high performers, shifting the focus from "self" to "service" can help them get started and stay consistent. When the idea of eating better or exercising feels daunting, reframing it as setting an example for others—your children, your team, or even your peers—can provide you with the motivation you need to get started. Other people are watching, and by modeling positive habits, you inspire them to do the same.

Take parents, for example. I've worked with many mothers who struggled to prioritize their own well-being. They felt guilty spending time on themselves. But when they reframed their self-care as a way to teach their children the value of health and balance, everything changed. Suddenly, it wasn't just about them—it was about being a leader in their own household.

The same is true in business and sports. Coaches, CEOs, and managers are all in positions of influence. If you're a coach who emphasizes discipline, commitment, and nutrition but fails to practice those values yourself, your message loses power.

You can't ask others to give their best if you're not modeling the same.

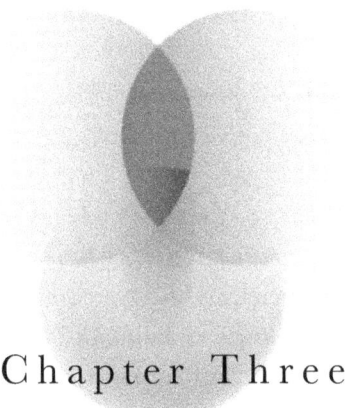

Chapter Three

A PURPOSEFUL SELF-CARE ROUTINE

UNFORTUNATELY, WE'VE ALL seen examples of people who set out to make some significant life change, but they couldn't keep it going for long. It's the New Year's resolution effect. For older people, this often happens because they get frustrated when they can't perform at the level they did in their twenties or thirties. They throw in the towel, thinking, *If I can't do what I used to, why bother at all?* This mindset, unfortunately, sabotages long-term health and growth and damages the example set for others.

But self-care isn't static. It evolves. What works for you today might not work in a decade, and that's OK. If you can't perform at the level you did in your twenties, that is perfectly fine. Your commitment to self-care can (and should) remain the same, even if the methods need to change. As Dr. Peter Attia often emphasizes that longevity is about adapting over time. The goal is to extend your *healthspan*—the years you live with vitality and productivity—not just your lifespan.[5]

Personally, while I can't do the same workouts I did in my wrestling days, I've adapted my routine. Recovery has become a bigger focus, and I've incorporated practices like stretching, mobility work, and mindful recovery techniques to maintain balance. This flexibility not only keeps me engaged but ensures that I'm building a model of self-care I can sustain for life.

Daily Self-Care Habits

One of the most powerful ways to build momentum for self-care is by *winning the morning*. I firmly believe the way you start your day sets the tone for everything that follows. But winning the morning actually starts the night before.

Sleep is the unsung hero of high performance. For years, I operated under the "sleep when you're dead" mentality. Burning the candle at both ends felt like the mark of ambition. But as I delved into the science, it became clear that sleep isn't optional—it's absolutely essential. Sleep restores balance to your nervous system, enhances cognitive function, and fuels your ability to attack the day.

To optimize sleep, I've worked hard on my *sleep hygiene*:
- **Dark Room:** Blackout curtains or a sleep mask to eliminate light.
- **Tech-Free Zone:** Turning off phones, TVs, and computers well before bedtime.
- **Consistent Routine:** Going to bed and waking up at the same time every day.

---

5   Peter Attia, *Outlive: The Science and Art of Longevity* (Scribner, 2022).

A PURPOSEFUL SELF-CARE ROUTINE

These small changes have made a big difference. I wake up with more energy and more drive to tackle my morning routine.

My morning routine, then, is simple but intentional. I start with movement—something as basic as stretching or a short walk. Movement wakes up the body and gets the blood flowing. From there, I often journal or reflect on my goals for the day (we'll talk more about journaling later). This practice aligns my mindset with my purpose and keeps me grounded.

In terms of nutrition, on most days, I opt for a high-protein, nutrient-dense breakfast that fuels my energy and keeps me sharp. And, yes, I hydrate. I'm a big believer in starting the day with water to rehydrate after sleep. Once or twice per week, I will fast in order to put my body in a state of ketosis. This has many health benefits, including burning fat for fuel during this period.

These small, consistent actions create a domino effect. When you start the day with wins, you're more likely to carry that momentum into everything else you do, and that sets a great example for those around you.

The next step in my morning routine is hydration. I'm a big believer in starting the day with *hydrogenated water*. You can make it at home using a generator or dissolve tablets into your water when traveling. Research suggests hydrogenated water has regenerative properties, promoting balance and recovery in the body.[6] It's my go-to before I even touch my first cup of coffee.

I won't lie—I *love* coffee. But I approach it with care. I enjoy a mushroom coffee blend from Four Sigmatic, which combines coffee with adaptogenic mushrooms like lion's mane and reishi.[7] This mix helps with mental clarity and focus without the jitters or crashes. I

---

6   International Journal of Molecular Sciences. "Potential Health Benefits of Hydrogen-Rich Water: A Systematic Review," accessed January 10, 2025, https://www.mdpi.com/1422-0067/25/2/973.
7   https://us.foursigmatic.com/collections/mushroom-coffee.

also make a point to cut off caffeine by 2:00 or 3:00 p.m. so it doesn't interfere with my sleep later.

When it's time for breakfast, I prioritize protein and steer clear of sugary, high-fat foods. My favorite go-to is protein pancakes. Here's the simple recipe:

- Sprouted oats
- Protein powder
- An egg
- A dash of mushroom powder
- Superfood powder for an extra boost

Blend them all together, cook it like a pancake, and top it with natural sweetness like fresh blueberries or a drizzle of honey. On simpler mornings, I'll opt for eggs and sourdough toast, but I'm mindful of keeping my insulin levels stable—no spiking my blood sugar first thing in the day.

Finally, movement is nonnegotiable in my morning routine, but I don't go all out. Mornings are for light, low-intensity activities: a brisk walk outside with my dog, stretching or mobility exercises, tidying up the house. I'm one of those people who can't leave the house without making the bed. It's like a mental "all-systems-go" signal for me.

Movement in the morning sets a physical and mental rhythm for the day ahead. By the time I've finished journaling, hydrating, fueling, and moving, I'm ready to dive into work. My mornings are when I'm most productive, so I tackle the day's priorities with focus. I aim to wrap up work by 3:00 or 3:30 p.m., following the principles from Tim Ferriss's *The 4-Hour Workweek*. While I haven't mastered that level of efficiency yet, I'm working toward it.

A PURPOSEFUL SELF-CARE ROUTINE

Finally, my evening routine is just as intentional as my morning routine. I focus on:
- Eating an early dinner (ideally before 7:00 p.m.) to avoid disrupting my sleep.
- Winding down with limited screen time.
- Preparing for restful sleep in a dark, quiet environment.

Good sleep is the secret weapon of high performance. It's when your body restores balance, your brain consolidates memories, and your energy regenerates. Without it, winning the morning—and the day—becomes an uphill battle.

Remember: This daily routine isn't just about checking boxes—it's about building momentum. It's a system that aligns the mind, body, and spirit for the day ahead. And it's adaptable. If I'm traveling, I adjust. If life throws me a curveball, I pivot. The key is consistency, not rigidity.

Winning the morning (and, therefore, the day) is a choice, and it starts the night before. When you set yourself up for success with intentional habits, you're not just improving your day—you're investing in your future. You are creating a rhythm of self-awareness, gratitude, and forward momentum that keeps you moving toward your goals. So grab your journal, pour yourself a glass of water (or hydrogenated water if you're feeling fancy), and start winning your mornings one small habit at a time.

Now, in my journey as a coach, teacher, and leader, I've come to realize that being intentional about how I structure my day is just as important as what I put on my plate or how many steps I take. With that in mind, let's look at some important tools that help me monitor and optimize my well-being.

Tactics and Tools to Optimize Self-Care

Sleep: Tracking Your Recharge

Sleep is the foundation of performance. To truly understand my sleep patterns, I use a device called *Whoop*. This wearable device tracks my sleep cycles, including deep sleep and REM sleep, and provides me with data that's invaluable for understanding how well my body is recovering. While no device is perfect, Whoop (and another excellent option, the *Oura Ring*) offers insights that are hard to ignore. For example, if my wearable reveals that I'm not getting enough restorative sleep, I know I'll be operating at a deficit the next day, so I can adjust accordingly.

When I first started using wearables years ago, I was fixated on tracking my workouts, but now I spend more time analyzing my sleep metrics than my training stats. Why? Because sleep sets the stage for everything else. Without quality rest, no amount of effort in the gym or the office is going to yield the results I'm after.

One other metric that I pay close attention to is my HRV, or heart rate variability. Without getting too deep into the weeds, HRV measures the changes in time between each heartbeat. It's a key indicator of how well the body balances between the **sympathetic nervous system** (the fight-or-flight response) and the **parasympathetic nervous system** (the rest-and-recover state).

A **higher HRV** suggests better adaptability, recovery, and overall resilience while a **lower HRV** can indicate stress, fatigue, or poor recovery. Tracking HRV is a valuable tool for understanding how well the body is managing stress and recovery, making it an important factor in achieving High Performance.

For those who prefer not to use wearables, I encourage my clients to keep a simple sleep journal. Record how long you slept, how you felt upon waking, and any factors that might have influenced your rest. Remember: Sleep is nonnegotiable if you want high performance.

TIME BLOCKING: THE SECRET WEAPON OF PRODUCTIVITY
One of the most impactful habits I've adopted is *time blocking*. This is a strategy that keeps me focused and ensures I'm making the most of my day. Here's how it works:
- **Break your day into chunks.** I typically set aside thirty-minute or fifteen-minute blocks for specific tasks, like answering emails, meeting with clients, or working on projects.
- **Stick to the plan.** Once the timer starts, I'm all in. No distractions. If I don't time block, I'm at risk of getting sidetracked, which easily becomes a rabbit hole of emails or random tasks that eat up hours if I'm not careful.
- **Close the loop.** I dedicate thirty minutes a day to emails, then shut it down. Endless email threads can become a productivity killer, so I try to handle them efficiently and move on.

By starting my day with a clear roadmap of priorities, I minimize stress and stay mentally sharp. This structure isn't rigid but intentional. And for someone like me who's easily distracted, it's a powerful tool for making progress.

CLOSING THE DAY
High performers don't just know how to work hard—they know when to stop. Early in my coaching career, I struggled with this. I would often stay up late grading papers, preparing lessons, or dealing with team issues, but eventually, I realized the cost. Pushing myself late into the night wasn't sustainable, and it stole from the next day's energy and performance.

These days, I set boundaries. By 6:00 or 7:00 p.m., I make a conscious effort to shut down work and shift into family mode. If something needs extra attention, I'll tackle it in the morning when my energy is higher. This practice of "closing the day" allows me to recharge mentally and emotionally so I show up fully for my family and for myself.

The evening isn't just downtime; it's recovery time. Transitioning from a work mindset to a relaxed state is important for balancing the nervous system. This is the time to reestablish parasympathetic balance, the "rest and digest" mode that helps counteract the stressors of the day.

Here are a few strategies that work for me:

- **Mindful entertainment:** I avoid overly stimulating TV shows. That means no murder mysteries or adrenaline-pumping dramas right before bed. Instead, I opt for something calming or light-hearted.
- **Family connection:** Spending time with loved ones, having meaningful conversations, or simply being present helps me decompress.
- **Presleep rituals:** Turning off screens, dimming the lights, and following a consistent bedtime routine all contribute to better sleep.

Self-care is about the long game. It's about finding a sustainable rhythm that aligns with your goals and values. Some days might require extra flexibility, and that's OK. But the key is to maintain your commitment to balance and recovery.

And self-care isn't selfish. Whether you're monitoring your sleep, blocking your time, or drawing boundaries between work and home life, every effort you make is an investment in your future and the future of all those people who look at your example. When you prioritize recovery and reflection, you'll find yourself better equipped to take on the challenges and opportunities that come your way.

Part Two

AWARENESS

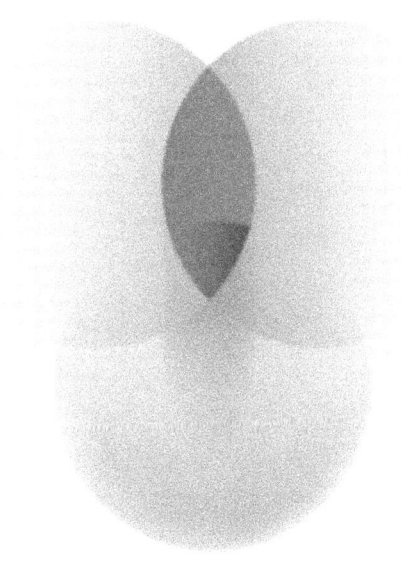

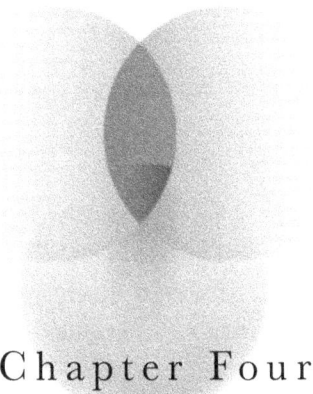

Chapter Four

BUILDING AWARENESS

AWARENESS IS WHERE everything begins. In the AOC model, it serves as the catalyst for growth and change. Without awareness, there's no clear starting point, and without a starting point, progress is impossible. Awareness is about understanding your current reality, examining the factors that influence your success, and then using that knowledge to set a direction for improvement.

Many people *believe* they are self-aware, but in practice, they struggle to see the full picture. They lack insight into how their habits, thoughts, relationships, and environments shape their outcomes. Through years of coaching and working with clients, I've learned that awareness requires more than mere observation. It demands active inquiry and the courage to confront uncomfortable truths about where you currently stand.

Two Dimensions of Awareness: Data and Reflection

Awareness has two dimensions: the *measurable* and the *intuitive* (i.e., *data* and *reflection*). Together, they create a full-spectrum understanding of where you are and what needs to change.

Hard data provides clarity. In health, these metrics might include your blood pressure, cholesterol levels, or step counts. In business, they could be revenue figures, customer satisfaction scores, or productivity metrics. These numbers offer an objective baseline that allows you to track where you stand and how you're progressing over time. But data is only valuable when paired with understanding. A cholesterol reading of 220, for example, is just a number until you interpret its implications. Does it signal a need for medication? Or is it an opportunity to make lifestyle changes? Effective awareness analyzes and applies the insights that the data provides.

The same principle applies in other areas of life. For athletes, win-loss records are straightforward, but digging deeper into performance trends often reveals actionable patterns. In business, financial reports tell a surface story, but understanding the underlying shifts, such as changes in customer behavior or operational efficiency, provides the real power.

Metrics tell part of the story, but true awareness also requires introspection. Self-reflection allows you to uncover the thoughts, feelings, and habits that shape your decisions. It asks deeper questions, such as, "What am I doing well? What's holding me back? Are my actions aligned with my values?"

Reflection is incredibly important because it reveals what numbers cannot—things like your motivations and blind spots. It helps you understand not just what is happening but also why. For example, you might notice that you skip workouts when your schedule feels tight, but reflection can uncover the underlying self-talk—"I'll never be consistent, so why bother?"—that keeps you stuck. Awareness of these patterns is the first step in breaking them.

Another important aspect of awareness is evaluating whether your daily actions reflect your stated values. A question I often pose to clients is, "What do you value most?" Common answers include family, health, or career success, but when we examine how they're spending their time, their schedules often tell a different story. This disconnect isn't uncommon, and it doesn't mean someone's values are insincere. Often, it's simply a lack of alignment between intentions and habits. Awareness helps bridge that gap. For example, if you value family but realize you're spending all your energy on work, awareness gives you the opportunity to adjust, perhaps by carving out intentional family time or delegating tasks at work.

Aligning your actions with your values doesn't just create consistency. It gives you a greater sense of fulfillment. When you live in alignment with what matters most, you create a sense of purpose and satisfaction that fuels further growth.

Awareness also means honestly identifying your strengths and weaknesses. While both strengths and weaknesses are important to understand, focusing on your strengths usually yields the greatest results. I once worked with a business owner who was an exceptional visionary, but he struggled with managing his team. By leaning into his strengths—in this case, strategy and long-term planning—we restructured his role to delegate day-to-day management. This not only improved his business but also increased his personal satisfaction.

The same principle applies to personal growth. Instead of obsessing over eliminating every weakness, focus on building habits that amplify your strengths. For example, if you're great at cooking healthy meals but struggle with regular exercise, start by enhancing your nutrition and let that momentum inspire changes in other areas.

This approach also works in reverse. Adding positive habits often crowds out negative ones. In nutrition, for example, focusing on incorporating more vegetables, lean proteins, and whole foods naturally reduces the consumption of less nutritious options. Similarly, focusing on strengths in other areas of life can help diminish the impact of your weaknesses.

AWARENESS IN PRACTICE

One daily practice I strongly encourage is *journaling*. It is one of the most effective tools for cultivating awareness because it provides a structured way to capture insights and track habits so you can reflect on your progress. A journal can help you monitor your health, assess your business ventures, or even explore your relationships. It acts as both a mirror and a map, showing you where you are and guiding you toward where you want to go.

For all of these reasons, journaling is a vital element of the AOC model. If you've never done it, or you're not quite comfortable with it, make it easy on yourself. Start by answering a simple question, such as, *Where am I today?* Without a clear baseline, it's impossible to grow. That's where journaling shines. It becomes your personal scoreboard, your accountability partner, and your coach all rolled into one.

Journaling is the first step in my morning routine because it gets my mind right from the very beginning and prepares me to face the day with purpose. First, it tracks the essentials: What am I eating and drinking? Did I get my workout in? What's my mood like today?

Second, it creates space for gratitude. Every morning, I jot down something I'm thankful for. Gratitude shifts your mindset from scarcity to abundance. For example, I might write about the joy of being a grandparent to eight incredible grandkids or the opportunity to watch my son coach wrestling. These small reflections add perspective and remind me why I show up every day.

BUILDING AWARENESS

If you're journaling at the end of the day, I suggest simple prompts like, "What went well today? What could I have done better? What am I grateful for?" Over time, daily reflections like these will reveal patterns, both positive and negative, that might otherwise go unnoticed. For example, many people don't realize how negative their inner dialogue is until they see it written down. Once identified, these thoughts can be replaced with empowering alternatives, creating a shift in mindset.

Another benefit of journaling is that it can easily become a daily habit. After all, awareness isn't a one-time exercise: It's a practice, and it requires ongoing reflection and a willingness to adapt as new information emerges. Whether you're using metrics to measure progress, journaling to explore your thoughts, or evaluating your alignment with your values, awareness equips you with the clarity to move forward with purpose.

It's not always comfortable to confront the truth about where you are, but it's incredibly important. Without awareness, you're essentially navigating life without a map. With it, you gain the direction and focus you need to take ownership of your journey and commit to meaningful change.

But awareness is more than knowing where you stand. It's also recognizing the hidden influences that shape your decisions, reactions, and outcomes. When you approach life with awareness, you're diving deep to uncover the beliefs and habits that drive your actions. This is not always comfortable work, but it's necessary for high performance in any area of life.

One of the biggest roadblocks to awareness is *personal bias*. We all come to the table with preconceived notions based on our experiences, the information we consume, and the narratives we've built about ourselves. These biases can be either empowering or limiting. For example, a belief like, "I've never been able to do this before, so

I'll probably fail again," can create a mental roadblock before you even begin. Recognizing these limiting beliefs is the first step in dismantling them.

Beyond merely *uncovering* the negative, awareness is also about understanding where your information comes from and ensuring that it's accurate. Are you relying on credible sources for your insights into health, fitness, or business? Are you engaging with books, mentors, and experts who challenge you to grow? Or are you stuck in an echo chamber that reinforces outdated or faulty ideas? By questioning your sources and being open to new perspectives, you can reshape your foundation for growth.

Mindfulness: The Gateway to Awareness

Achieving awareness means learning to be present. Too often, we live in the future, worrying about what might happen, or in the past, rehashing what we could have done differently. While both perspectives can offer valuable lessons, they can also distract us from the here and now. True awareness happens in the present moment when you're fully engaged with what's happening right now.

Practicing mindfulness can help you cultivate this presence. Simple tools like deep breathing, meditation, or visualization exercises can ground you in the moment and help you assess your current state without judgment. But mindfulness isn't a skill you can summon on demand. Like any skill, it requires regular practice. Just as an athlete trains consistently to perfect a move, practicing daily mindfulness prepares you to use it effectively during critical moments.

For example, when I first began coaching athletes, I encouraged them to use visualization techniques right before a competition. The result, however, was frustration and anxiety because they hadn't practiced these skills regularly. It was like asking them to master a complex wrestling move without ever drilling it in practice. Over time, I learned that mindfulness tools must become part of your daily routine to be effective when you need them most.

Focusing on the present is important because it contributes to *situational awareness*, which is your ability to respond effectively in the moment. High performers excel in this area, particularly under pressure. They manage deadlines, navigate critical decisions, and adapt to high-stakes scenarios with composure. Situational awareness isn't just about reacting to things as they happen but recognizing your emotional and physiological state in the moment and using that insight to perform at your best.

When discussing situational awareness, it's important to understand the *performance anxiety curve*. This psychological principle suggests that a certain level of anxiety can enhance your performance by sharpening focus and driving effort. However, too much anxiety pushes you over the curve, which leads to diminished performance and potential burnout.

Managing this balance is a hallmark of high performers. Athletes like Patrick Mahomes demonstrate incredible situational awareness by staying calm and collected under immense pressure. Studies using wearables like the Whoop device are beginning to shed light on how elite performers maintain physiological and mental control during these high-pressure moments. As it turns out, high performance isn't about eliminating anxiety altogether but channeling it effectively.

For most of us, achieving this balance requires strategies like mindfulness, breath work, or even reframing the situation to reduce its perceived intensity. Whether you're preparing for a big presentation or facing a tight deadline, learning to manage situational awareness can transform stress into a catalyst for success.

Awareness Lays the Foundation

Awareness doesn't exist in isolation. It's the foundation for the next steps in the AOC model: ownership and commitment. You can't own your challenges or commit to meaningful change if you're not first aware of where you stand. Awareness provides the feedback you need to identify blind spots and adjust your approach so you can set actionable goals. By questioning your biases, practicing mindfulness, and seeking feedback from both hard data and trusted relationships, you can cultivate a deeper understanding of yourself and your environment. This clarity not only sets the stage for personal transformation but also equips you to handle life's challenges with resilience and confidence.

Whether you're aiming for personal growth, professional success, healthier relationships, or better health, awareness is where the journey begins. It's the lens through which you see every other step: Be present, be curious, and watch as your self-awareness unlocks new possibilities. Indeed, awareness is the key to transformation because it helps you see yourself clearly and recognize your impact on others. That makes it the first step in any meaningful change, as well as a powerful tool for shaping your relationships, career, and overall performance.

One of the most overlooked aspects of awareness is how we are perceived by others. While we can't fully read minds, there are clues all around us in nonverbal communication, the tone of conversations, and how people respond to us. Are people engaged when you speak? Or are they cutting off conversations or avoiding interaction altogether? This feedback, subtle as it may be, is invaluable. Being attuned to these signals helps you understand how you're showing up in the world and where you might need to adjust.

Remember: This isn't just about self-improvement for its own sake. Relationships, both personal and professional, thrive when we're mindful of how our words and actions land with others. If you notice patterns, like people pulling back or conflicts arising, it's a sign that you need to reflect. And that reflection naturally segues into ownership, the next pillar of the AOC model, as you acknowledge your role and make changes to bridge any gaps in how you're perceived versus how you want to be.

Consistent and Continuous Learning

Awareness is a commitment to consistently observe your behaviors and patterns. That's why journaling is such an effective way to cultivate this habit. By documenting your actions, thoughts, and routines, you begin to notice recurring patterns, both the good and the bad. I encourage clients to block out time during the day to jot down what they're doing and how they're feeling. This can be as granular as tracking habits every fifteen to thirty minutes or simply noting major events and their impact. Over time, patterns emerge. A behavior that happens sporadically might not be significant, but something that occurs daily or weekly could be a sign of a habit that's worth paying attention to.

Awareness also helps you evaluate habits more objectively. Is a certain routine driving positive results? Great, lean into it. On the other hand, if a behavior repeatedly causes stress or negative outcomes, that's an opportunity to either eliminate or replace it. For many, replacing a bad habit with a positive one is more effective than simply trying to cut out the bad behavior. The idea is to gradually crowd out the negative with constructive actions.

Of course, your environment plays a massive role in shaping your behavior and performance. This includes both the physical spaces you inhabit and the people you surround yourself with. According to Jim Rohn, you are the average of the five people you spend the most time with. If those people are encouraging and growth-oriented, you're likely to rise to their level. But if your environment is filled with negativity or complacency, it's much harder to stay motivated and grow.

The balance of your network is key. Ideally, you're in the middle, learning from those who are ahead of you while mentoring those who can benefit from your experience. This dynamic creates a cycle of accountability and mutual support. Importantly, this isn't a rigid structure. Different people may serve these roles in different areas of your life. Someone who mentors you in your career might turn to you for advice on fitness or relationships. The goal is to create a network that fosters growth in all aspects of your life.

Above all, bear in mind that awareness isn't static. Rather, it's a skill that grows with practice and intentionality. One of the most effective ways to deepen awareness is by staying curious and committed to learning. Reading books, listening to podcasts, and engaging in meaningful conversations are all ways to expand your perspective and challenge your thinking.

In addition to seeking knowledge from external sources, it's equally important to engage with your "soft network," the trusted people in your life who can offer honest feedback and help you see your blind spots. These aren't just casual acquaintances but the individuals who truly understand your goals and can provide valuable insights into your strengths, weaknesses, and opportunities for growth.

By combining external resources (books, courses, data) with internal reflection and meaningful conversations, you create a robust system for cultivating awareness. This practice not only helps you identify areas for improvement but also equips you to handle challenges with greater clarity and confidence.

Awareness is powerful, but it requires consistency to create lasting change. It's not enough to reflect once and move on. You need to build a habit of regularly evaluating where you are and where you're headed. Track your actions, revisit your goals regularly, and check in with your environment and relationships. Stay present. Awareness thrives in the here and now, not in the past or the distant future. Again, while reflection on past experiences can be valuable, it's easy to get stuck replaying regrets or projecting fears. True awareness comes from engaging fully with the moment, including your current state, and using that knowledge to make intentional choices.

In the end, awareness is both a lens and a foundation. It helps you see yourself and your surroundings more clearly while laying the groundwork for meaningful change. Whether you're working to improve relationships, advance your career, or enhance your well-being, awareness is the starting point. Acknowledge where you are, be open to feedback, and embrace the process of growth. With awareness, you're not just reacting to life—you're shaping it.

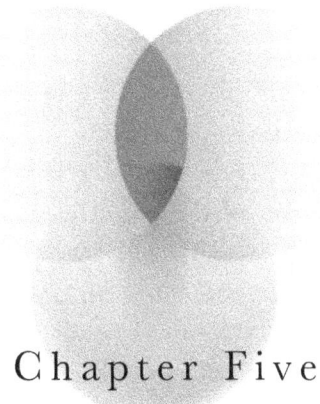

Chapter Five

DEEPENING AWARENESS

DEEPENING YOUR AWARENESS (of yourself, your behavior patterns, surroundings, relationships, etc.) requires curiosity and courage. It's challenging at times, but the rewards—better decisions, stronger relationships, and a clearer sense of purpose—are profound. The more aware you become, the more empowered you will be to create a fulfilling and successful life for yourself and others.

It can be helpful to have others on the journey. As a coach, I've always believed in practicing what I preach. That's why I've consistently sought out coaches and mentors to guide me—not just in my professional life but in my personal growth as well. From business coaches to fitness trainers, these individuals have offered insights that I couldn't have uncovered on my own. To grow, you need people who challenge your perspective, whether they're paid professionals or trusted mentors. The truth is, no matter how much success you've achieved, having someone help you see your blind spots and avoid potential missteps is extremely valuable.

This mindset applies to everyone. Growth isn't a solo journey. We all need to seek guidance, ask thoughtful questions, and stay open to feedback, even when it's uncomfortable. Personal development thrives on curiosity. When we approach our habits and emotions with a sense of wonder, we ignite the motivation to explore and improve.

Curiosity naturally leads to engagement. In my experience, clients who ask the most questions, whether about their health, work, relationships, or something else, tend to stay motivated. Their curiosity becomes the driving force behind their progress.

If you're wondering how to cultivate this curiosity, start simple. Ask yourself questions like *Why did I react this way in that situation? What is the underlying cause of my behavior? How could I approach this differently in the future?*

Once you understand your reactions and motivations, you create space for ownership and commitment. And as we said in the previous chapter, journaling and mindfulness provide powerful tools for doing this. Writing down your thoughts can help you uncover patterns, while mindfulness encourages you to observe without judgment.

SEEING PAST YOUR BLIND SPOTS

Your blind spots can hinder your progress, but in many cases, these blind spots are areas of behavior or thinking that we don't even recognize as problematic. This is why feedback is so important. Surround yourself with people who provide constructive observations while staying mindful of whose opinions you value. Too much input, especially from unqualified sources, can lead to overwhelm.

Cognitive biases also pose a challenge. Preconceived notions and confirmation bias can distort our perception of reality, making it harder to grow. It's important to recognize these biases and question your own assumptions. Don't settle for "I already know how to do this." Instead, ask, "What could I learn from this situation?"

Distractions further complicate awareness. In today's fast-paced world, multitasking often feels like a necessity, but science has shown that multitasking isn't the brain's strength—it's just rapid task-switching, which actually diminishes productivity and focus. Time blocking, scheduling, and limiting interruptions like email can help you maintain the concentration you need for growth.

One of the greatest barriers to awareness, however, is the *fear of facing the truth*. Many people avoid self-assessment because they're afraid of what they might find. I've encountered this countless times, whether through my work at a wellness center or conversations with clients. People shy away from knowing their cholesterol levels, their spending habits, or even their emotional struggles because the truth feels overwhelming. But here's the thing: Awareness is just information. It's not inherently good or bad. It's what you do with it that matters. Instead of viewing uncomfortable truths as negatives, reframe them as opportunities for growth. Whether it's a bad habit, a poor decision, an unhealthy relationship, or a tough situation, acknowledging it is the first step toward meaningful change.

I once spoke to a woman on a flight who confessed she avoided self-reflection because she feared discovering "who she really was." This fear kept her stuck. But, as I told her, you can't move forward without knowing where you *really* are today. Facing the truth isn't about judgment but empowerment. When you reframe discomfort as a chance to grow, it becomes a powerful catalyst for change.

Whether you're seeking feedback, journaling, self-reflecting, or questioning your assumptions, every step you take deepens your understanding and moves you closer to your goals. Embrace the process, face the truth, and stay curious. The rewards of this journey are worth it.

Movement and Motivation

Bear in mind, just as it is possible to have *too little* information (about yourself, your environment, etc.), you can also have *too much*. You can be overwhelmed by information just as easily as you can be paralyzed by a lack of it. In fact, "paralysis by analysis" is common in today's world, where we're inundated with data and decisions. The key to breaking free is *movement*.

Contrary to the idea that motivation fuels action, it's often the reverse. Action usually sparks motivation. When we're stagnant, overthinking takes over, and awareness can feel out of reach. However, by simply creating movement—whether it's a walk, a bike ride, or any low-level physical activity—we can unlock new perspectives and ideas.

Some of my most creative moments happen during periods of light activity, what we previously called "Zone 2 training." So I'm not talking about pushing your limits or maxing out your endurance. This is about gentle, sustainable movement that allows your mind to wander and engage. For me, morning walks or leisurely bike rides are ideal times for creative breakthroughs. These moments help open mental gateways, providing clarity and fostering awareness in ways that sitting still often can't.

Awareness is about understanding your mental and emotional state, but at the same time, it's also about being in tune with your physical self. As we said, modern tools like wearable fitness devices can provide valuable, actionable feedback about your body in real time. For example, days when my wearable shows I've been in a constant state of high alert, indicating prolonged sympathetic activation, are rarely my most creative or insightful days. While I might get a lot of tasks done, those aren't the moments when I'm fostering instinct, insight, or deeper awareness. On the other hand, when my metrics show a balance between activity and rest, I find myself more reflective, innovative, and attuned to my surroundings.

DEEPENING AWARENESS

Visualization is another powerful tool for awareness. By mentally walking through scenarios, you can gain clarity about your goals, obstacles, and potential outcomes. This practice enhances your ability to recognize patterns and anticipate challenges, making it an important part of any high performer's toolkit.

Gratitude also plays a significant role in developing awareness. Taking time to appreciate your progress or even small victories can ground you in the present moment, enhancing your perspective and reducing the overwhelm that can come from focusing solely on what's ahead.

Finally, it's important to understand that awareness is not a passive state. *Awareness is something you must actively cultivate.* Whether through movement, mindfulness, visualization, or leveraging modern technology, the goal is to create a consistent practice of tuning into yourself. Awareness sets the foundation for ownership, the next critical step on the journey to high performance.

With that in mind, let's transition to the concept of ownership—taking what you've learned about yourself and using it to create meaningful change. But remember: Awareness is where it all begins. Without it, you can't truly move forward.

Part Three

OWNERSHIP

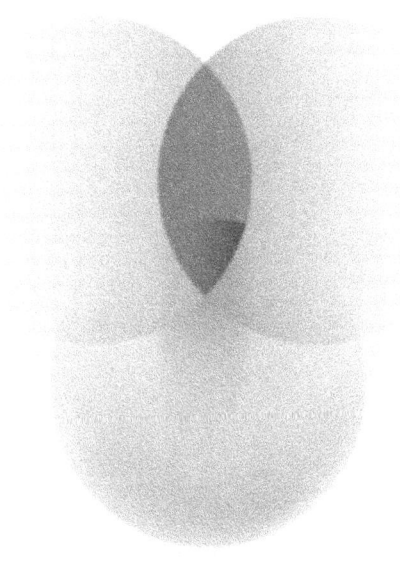

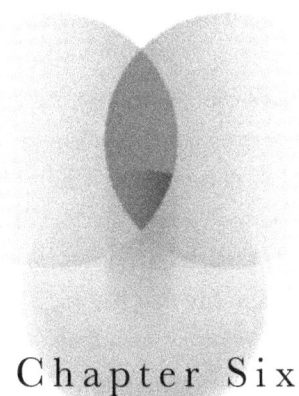

Chapter Six

TAKING RESPONSIBILITY

GROWING UP, I got an early lesson in ownership. My dad was an entrepreneur who owned multiple businesses, and he showed me what it looks like to truly take responsibility. Even as a young kid, I saw it in the way he handled personnel, financial challenges, and the daily grind of running a business. He was the workhorse of the family operation. He rarely took sick days, and we never went on spontaneous vacations.

The only trips we took as a family were once-a-year drives to St. Louis to catch a Cardinals game. Those rare moments, such as watching Bob Gibson and the 1967 starting lineup, were more than just fun. They were my first glimpse into the sacrifice and dedication it takes to own something fully.

These early experiences taught me that ownership isn't just a title or a piece of paper. It's about stepping up and being fully accountable for your outcomes. That's why ownership became the cornerstone of my AOC model. Without ownership, nothing else works.

Ownership *starts* with taking responsibility for your actions and the outcomes they produce. When I work with people, I often see a tendency to deflect. If their health numbers are off, the first thing they'll say is, "It's genetics. My dad had high cholesterol." Sure, genetics play a role, but if you don't own the issue, you can't fix it. The same principle applies in business. If you're not owning your role in the numbers, processes, or outcomes, you're stuck. But ownership isn't just about fixing the negatives. It's also about celebrating the successes that come from the effort you've put in.

In sports, coaches don't just focus on wins and losses. When teams are heading into playoffs or championships, they talk about the work that got them there—the practices, the sacrifices, the hard work, the grind. The same is true in life. Whether you're looking at personal health, business performance, or relationships, you have to own the actions that led you to where you are. The results are just the byproduct of that effort.

Ownership is deeply tied to resilience. When you take responsibility for your outcomes, you're better equipped to bounce back when things go wrong. High performers tend to have this mindset. They own their mistakes, learn from them, and pivot. On the other hand, people who lack resilience often get stuck in negative loops, blaming others and repeating the same behaviors over and over again. Resilience is about breaking that cycle and saying, "This is my responsibility, and I'm going to fix it."

That doesn't mean you have to take on the weight of the world. Part of ownership is understanding what you can control and letting go of what you can't. Trying to fix everything will only lead to burnout. Instead, the idea is to focus on what's within your power to change.

This is actually one of the most empowering aspects of ownership, realizing it's all yours—the good, the bad, and the ugly. It's not your spouse's fault, your boss's fault, or your coworker's fault. Once you stop pointing fingers, you're free to act. As a coach, I've walked into tough situations where it would've been easy to blame the previous leadership or a lack of resources, but the moment you take ownership, you start seeing opportunities instead of obstacles.

You are stepping into the driver's seat of your life, taking responsibility for where you are, celebrating your wins, and learning from your failures. When you own your journey, you create space to grow, pivot, and succeed. So the challenge is simple: *Own it*. The good, the bad, and everything in between. Once you do, you'll be amazed at what you're capable of achieving.

Four Steps to Owning Your Journey

When it comes to creating real, lasting change in your life, ownership is what makes it all possible. It's the linchpin of the AOC model, and it's where everything starts to click. But what does owning your journey actually look like in practice? Let me break it down into four practical steps that can supercharge your path to growth and success.

1. Set Your Own Goals

When it comes to goal setting, you need to do more than merely write down a wish list of things you hope to accomplish. You need to make those goals truly *yours*. When your goals come from the outside, whether from a company, a coach, parents, or even a well-meaning friend, they lack the power of personal buy-in. Think about it. When a company dictates goals to employees without their input, it's no wonder those goals fail to ignite any passion. The same goes for a coach declaring championship aspirations without team involvement.

Your goals need to reflect *your* desires and *your* vision. Writing them down is a good place to start, but it doesn't end there. Track your progress toward achieving them in a journal. Set deadlines. Reflect on your milestones. By owning your goals, you give yourself the power to execute them with conviction.

2. Reflect on Your Choices

Life is a series of choices, big and small. Ownership means pausing to ask, "Why did I make that choice? Was it intentional, or was I just going through the motions?" Far too often, people live mindlessly, making decisions out of habit or convenience rather than purpose.

For example, why did you reach for a sugary snack this morning instead of starting your day with a healthy breakfast? Winning the morning sets the tone for the day. If you're not mindful of your decisions, you risk falling into patterns that work against you. Reflecting on your choices, both the good and the bad, creates awareness. It's like shining a flashlight on your habits and understanding what's really driving them.

3. Learn from Your Failures

Failure isn't final unless you let it be. In my coaching career, I've seen countless athletes, officials, and professionals face setbacks. As long as you're still lacing up your shoes, figuratively or literally, you're still in the game.

There's a powerful tradition in wrestling where retiring athletes place their shoes on the mat after their final competition. It's a ceremonial goodbye, a way of saying, "This chapter is complete." But until that moment, the athlete is still learning, growing, and giving their best.

Failures are mere stepping stones. They're lessons in disguise. If you're willing to own your mistakes and adapt, you'll keep moving forward. It's only when you give up and stop trying that failure becomes permanent.

4. Create an Accountability-Rich Environment

As I previously mentioned, you are the average of the five people you spend the most time with. The company you keep can make or break your journey. Beyond tracking your own progress, you also need to create an environment that fosters growth. Who are your friends? Who are your peers? Are they pushing you to be better, or are they holding you back?

The beauty of ownership is that you get to choose your environment. You can surround yourself with people who inspire and challenge you to grow. One of the reasons I love the communities I'm part of, like the coaching world or my professional networks, is that they're rich with opportunities for personal and professional development. Whether it's engaging with thought leaders on LinkedIn or mentoring high school athletes, I'm constantly learning and growing, even as I help others learn and grow.

In my work with high performance individuals, whether in wellness, fitness, or business, one thing stands out: These people are motivated to grow. They're not content with mediocrity. They've chosen environments that support them and help them level up. And let me tell you, being surrounded by people with that kind of drive is hugely significant.

When I look at my own life, I see how important it has been to intentionally place myself in what I call "rich environments." These are spaces where growth is not just possible but inevitable. My wife and I made it a priority to immerse ourselves in such communities, and now I see my children doing the same. They've watched us choose to connect with people who inspire us, attend events that expand our horizons, and seek out experiences that push us forward.

The truth is, no one hands you a blueprint for this. No teacher in high school or college says, "Here's how to build a life that fosters personal and professional growth." Sure, schools train you for jobs, but they rarely equip you with the tools to create a rich life beyond that. You're not taught how to pick the right conventions to attend, the right mentors to seek out, or the right people to surround yourself with. That part is up to you.

If you don't create your environment, someone else will do it for you. And when that happens, you're no longer steering your own ship. You're just a passenger in someone else's plan. So take charge of the spaces you inhabit and make sure they align with your goals and values.

Building a System for Success

If you're part of a football team, it's easy to say, "We didn't win because the team as a whole didn't perform." But what was your specific role in that outcome? Maybe you were a defensive tackle. Did you give it your all? Did you show up prepared? Did you take responsibility for your part in the collective effort?

The same principle applies in business. If your company isn't growing the way it should, it's tempting to blame external factors such as the market, the economy, or even your coworkers. But what was your part in that puzzle? Did you bring your best ideas to the table? Did you take ownership of your responsibilities?

Ownership doesn't just happen. You have to intentionally create systems and methods that keep you accountable and help you grow. That means actively seeking out those rich environments and committing to showing up in them.

Choose the right people: Who you surround yourself with matters. Are your friends and colleagues pushing you to be better, or are they holding you back?

Seek out opportunities: Attend that conference, join that mastermind group, or take that class. Even if it's not directly in your field, it could spark the growth you didn't know you needed.

Stay mindful: Be intentional about your choices. Reflect on how your decisions—big and small—are shaping your path.

At the end of the day, ownership is about owning *everything*. Your growth, your setbacks, your role in the bigger picture—it's all on you. When you take ownership, you gain the power to create the outcomes you want. No one else is going to do it for you, but that's the beauty of it. You get to write your own story. So, why not make it a great one?

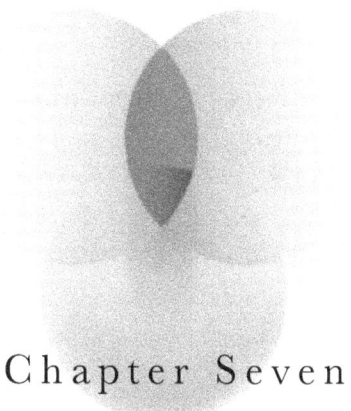

Chapter Seven

OVERCOMING BARRIERS TO OWNERSHIP

NOW, LET'S MOVE beyond just your goals and environment. You also need to take ownership of your *thoughts* and the way you talk to yourself. It's easy to overlook how much the words you hear and say, both consciously and unconsciously, shape your reality. This is the core of neurolinguistic programming, or as it's often called today, *neurolinguistic conditioning*. It's all about how our brain (neuro) interacts with language (linguistic) to influence our behavior and beliefs (conditioning).

The problem is most of us are running scripts in our heads that sabotage our potential. The noise of social media, our past failures and regrets, and even well-meaning criticism pile up over the years to convince us that we're not good enough or not deserving. These negative scripts create mental roadblocks that hold us back from reaching our full potential.

Ownership begins when you decide to rewrite the script. That means reclaiming the narrative in your mind and shifting from "I'm not good enough" to "I am capable. I am resilient. I can handle this." At first, this new script might feel forced, but over time, these positive affirmations will reshape your mindset and give you the confidence to act.

A Mindset for Action

Once you're thinking differently, you need to start acting differently, too. The way I approach this is with three simple but powerful statements:

- **I am.** Affirm who you are and what you're capable of. "I am disciplined. I am someone who gets things done. I am capable of handling challenges." These statements lay the foundation for a strong self-image.
- **I do.** Ownership requires action. "I do the work. I do show up for myself and others. I do prioritize my goals." This shifts the focus from intention to execution.
- **I have control.** While you can't control everything, there are things firmly within your grasp. "I have control over my attitude, my effort, and my responses to challenges." Owning what you can control and letting go of what you can't is empowering.

When you start with "I am," reinforce it with "I do," and focus on "I have control," you build a loop of positive belief and action. This rewriting of your inner script isn't a one-time event. It must become a daily commitment. Each morning, remind yourself, "I am capable, I do the work, and I have control over my attitude and effort today." Write these affirmations down if it helps.

Think about how you handle setbacks. Instead of spiraling into self-doubt, ask yourself, *What can I control here? How can I respond in a way that reflects my best self?* You're not just reacting to circumstances but actively deciding how you'll show up. This not only helps you hit your goals but also builds resilience. When you take ownership of your thoughts and actions, you empower yourself to keep going even when things get tough. I'm not suggesting that you should pretend everything is perfect. Rather, it's about saying, "This is my life, my challenge, and my opportunity to grow."

Ownership isn't something anyone can give you. You must claim it for yourself. Once you do, you will stop waiting for circumstances to line up and start creating the life you want. It all starts with that decision to rewrite your script and own your outcomes.

You choose your own path. No one else determines your direction—you do. Every decision you make is a reflection of your ownership, shaping your experiences and outcomes. When you embrace this mindset, you acknowledge that your path is yours to design, commit to, and ultimately accept the outcomes of, whether positive or negative.

Now, let's be real. Not every outcome will be solely yours. Life often involves teamwork and collective efforts. But even in those scenarios, taking ownership of your role within the bigger picture is important. Take leadership as an example. The best leaders own the results, good or bad. When their team wins, they credit the whole group, but when there's a loss, they shoulder their own responsibility. Behind closed doors, hard conversations might happen to address mistakes, but publicly, the leader owns it. This creates a culture where others feel supported and willing to take ownership themselves.

Owning your mistakes is just as important as owning your successes. Whether it's a misstep in business, sports, or a personal decision, the most successful people acknowledge where they fell short and learn from it. They don't point fingers at others—they take responsibility.

And by owning their mistakes, they position themselves to grow and improve.

You need to not only recognize a problem but also take responsibility to fix it. Sometimes, that means tapping into your own creativity and skills. Other times, it means asking for help. Yes, asking for help is a form of ownership! You don't have to do everything yourself. In fact, quite the opposite. High performers recognize that they don't have all the answers or tools, but they *own* the responsibility to seek out people who can help. Whether it's a mentor, a peer, a friend, or even AI technology, leveraging resources is a powerful way to create solutions.

You also need to set healthy boundaries. If you don't value your own time, energy, and focus, you'll struggle to maintain the level of performance you want. That means saying yes to the right things. By aligning your actions with your priorities, you ensure that your effort is spent on what truly matters. Think of boundaries as a filter. They help you separate what's important from what's just noise. Without them, you risk spreading yourself too thin and losing sight of your goals. High performers don't try to do everything—they focus on doing the *right* things with excellence.

Reflect, Improve, and Stay True

As we said earlier, ownership requires constant reflection and improvement. Just because something worked yesterday doesn't mean it will work tomorrow. Success isn't a static achievement but a dynamic process. The best performers debrief after every competition or project and ask themselves, *What worked? What didn't? How can I improve?*

This reflective mindset ensures that you're always adapting and growing. Whether it's a sports team analyzing a win or loss, a business revisiting a marketing campaign, or an individual reevaluating their daily habits, the goal is the same: *to keep evolving and adapting.*

Remember: True ownership aligns your actions with your values. If what you're working toward doesn't resonate with your priorities, it's time to reassess. There's no point in pouring effort into something that doesn't matter to you. Stephen Covey said it best: "It's one thing to be busy; it's another to be busy with purpose." So take a step back and ask yourself, *Are my efforts aligned with what I truly value? Am I climbing the right ladder?*

Ultimately, by owning every part of your journey in this way, you naturally move ownership into the next part of the AOC model: commitment. You're recognizing what's in your control and acknowledging the outcomes, and then you're stepping up and saying, "I am going to commit fully."

Committing to something is an act of ownership in itself. It's drawing a line in the sand and saying, "This is mine, and I'm going all in." Whether it's a decision to improve your health, focus on your career, or strengthen your relationships, ownership is what gets you to the starting line. Commitment is what keeps you in the race. With that in mind, we'll take a look at the role commitment plays in a high-performing lifestyle.

Part Four

COMMITMENT

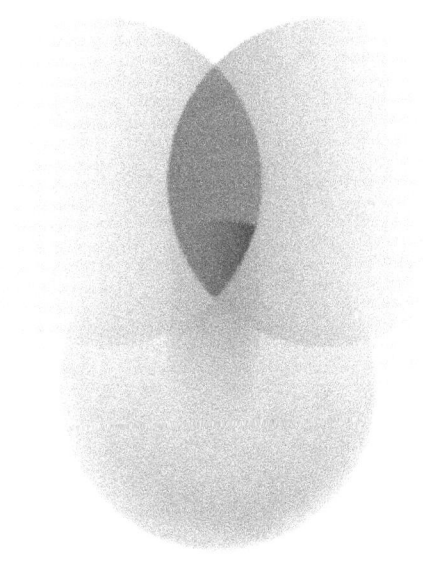

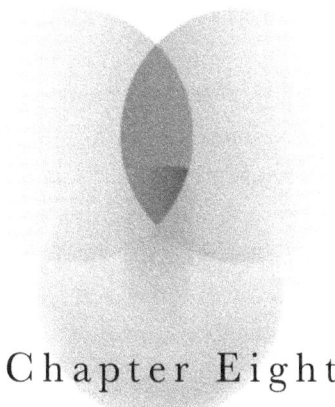

Chapter Eight

PRIORITIZING ACTION OVER MOTIVATION

IN THE AOC model, awareness, ownership, and commitment, each part plays an important role, but commitment is where everything comes alive. You master awareness by understanding your landscape, resources, and skills. You embrace ownership by taking full responsibility for your actions and outcomes. But without commitment, nothing moves forward. It's the engine that turns plans into progress.

Once you've laid the groundwork with awareness and ownership, commitment is where you roll up your sleeves and make it happen. Every big win starts with a single step. Build momentum through consistent actions, and bigger achievements will follow. Science supports this, with experts like Dr. Andrew Huberman emphasizing the importance of small victories. As he puts it, "Small actions, done consistently, lead to profound changes in your brain and body."[8]

Each win, no matter how minor, fuels your confidence and keeps you moving forward. Setting your alarm for 6:00 a.m. and actually getting out of bed when it rings might not seem like much, but it's a win. That one step leads to another and another, and before you know it, you're building habits that stick.

Small wins aren't just psychological fluff. They create momentum for bigger achievements. In business, a small win might be streamlining your finances or delegating a key task. In fitness, it could be showing up for a short workout. For relationships, it might mean taking the time for an intentional conversation. These steps might seem minor, but they add up in meaningful ways.

Consistency is the key ingredient in commitment. In a world obsessed with instant gratification, simply showing up every day consistently is a superpower. Small, steady actions compound over time, creating results that would have seemed impossible in the beginning. Think of it like a faucet dripping water into a glass. Each drop is small, but eventually, the glass fills. Turn off the faucet, and progress stops. Keep it dripping, and you'll reach your goal.

Staying consistent doesn't mean avoiding failure. High performers understand that failure is part of the process. What sets them apart is their willingness to keep going, even when things get tough. They understand that commitment isn't about perfection but persistence.

The beauty of commitment is that it builds on itself. Start with small wins. Be consistent. Focus on what matters most. Over time, those small steps create big changes. This is where intention becomes transformation and where high performance takes root.

---

8 Dr. Andrew Huberman, host, *Huberman Lab*, podcast, "How to Focus to Change Your Brain," October 3, 2022, https://www.hubermanlab.com/episode/how-to-focus-to-change-your-brain.

Of course, not everything in life requires 100 percent commitment, and that's OK. We all have things we enjoy but aren't ready to pour all of our time and energy into—and that's perfectly healthy. For example, I love to golf. It's a passion of mine, and I get so much joy from being out on the course. But I also have to own the fact that I'm not willing to commit five or six hours a day to become a great golfer. That's not where my priorities lie. I enjoy golf, but it doesn't rank in my top five priorities.

You don't have to give every hobby or activity your all. What you do have to do is identify the things that truly matter to you—your top three, four, or five priorities—and commit to those fully. For some, those priorities might include faith, family, career, health, or personal growth. For others, it could look completely different. The point is that those priorities are yours to define. What matters most to you? What are you willing to say, "This is worth my full effort?"

By taking ownership of your commitments, you can focus your energy on the areas that align with your values and goals. When you commit fully to those priorities, you're laying the groundwork for real growth and meaningful success. Remember this: *Owning your commitments is a choice.* It's saying, "This is mine, and I'm willing to do what it takes." And when you make that choice, you set yourself up for a life filled with purpose, progress, and high performance.

THE POWER OF BLIND FAITH

Fortunately, commitment doesn't have to be an all-out sprint toward quick success or immediate results. You're probably not going to win a state championship or land a major business deal overnight. Instead, success comes from a slow, steady drip of effort over time. And sometimes, that drip requires taking a leap of faith, believing that even when you don't see immediate progress, it's all going to pay off.

Blind faith is an underrated part of the commitment equation. As a coach, I've often had to instill belief and confidence in people who couldn't yet see success for themselves. I'll never forget a young wrestler I coached named Jason High. As a youth wrestler, Jason's record was one win and thirteen losses—hardly a confidence booster. When he joined our high school program as a freshman, his frustration was palpable. I remember one conversation midway through his first season when Jason looked me in the eye and said, "Coach, I was one-and-thirteen last year. Why would anyone think I'll ever be any good at this?"

That was the moment for blind faith. I told Jason, "You have to trust the process. You've got the athleticism, and there were so many reasons for your struggles before—maturity, circumstances, timing—but none of that defines what you can become. If you drip into this process every single day, success will come. I can't promise exactly what it'll look like, but the formula works. Awareness, ownership, and commitment will get you there."

And we both owned it. I committed to providing him with the tools, training partners, and guidance he needed to improve. Jason committed to showing up and working hard every day, no matter how tough it got. Fast forward a few years, and that same kid went from barely making the varsity team to becoming a state placer his senior year. He then wrestled at a junior college before transferring to the University of Nebraska to compete at the NCAA level.

It wasn't magic. It was the power of consistent effort—dripping into the process day by day. Jason transformed as an athlete, and he became living proof of how small wins, compounded over time, create big results.

Movement Fuels Motivation

A critical piece of this commitment puzzle is understanding the relationship between movement and motivation. Most people believe motivation is something that strikes like lightning—a sudden surge of inspiration that propels us into action. But the truth is, motivation isn't what gets you moving. Actually, it's the reverse. Movement is what brings motivation.

Picture this scene. It's a lazy afternoon, and you've planned to work out. You're slouched on the couch, waiting for a magical burst of energy to get you up. But it's never coming. Motivation isn't going to knock on your door. What *will* get you moving is movement. Get moving. Get off the couch, grab your workout shoes, or pack your gym bag. That tiny action creates momentum, and before you know it, you're lacing up and out the door. This is how motivation really works. As it turns out, *motivation is a byproduct of taking action.* High performers don't wait for motivation—they create it. They know that movement leads to momentum, and momentum generates motivation. It's a cycle that starts with one simple step.

Of course, commitment also demands resilience. You must develop the ability to stay dedicated even when things don't go as planned. To do that, you need to be fully invested, remaining loyal to your goals and finding ways to keep going, even when progress feels slow.

Motivation doesn't always come naturally, and setbacks will test your resolve, but with resilience, you can push through those moments because you understand that success isn't always linear and that every step, no matter how small, contributes to the bigger picture.

As I always tell my athletes, *you don't have to see the finish line to believe it's there.* Start with what you can control—your effort, your attitude, and your willingness to take one more step. Drip into the process, have faith, and let those small wins stack up. Whether you're chasing athletic excellence, business success, better relationships, or personal growth, the formula is the same: commit fully, stay consistent, and trust the journey.

Resilience + Grit = An Unshakable Foundation

Resiliency is the glue that keeps your goals intact, even when the outcomes aren't immediately favorable. For me, this means reframing setbacks. It's not about brushing failures aside or pretending they didn't happen but learning from them. In fact, I often write about my worst days in my gratitude journal because those are the days I've grown the most.

When I talk to teams or clients, I ask them, "Who here has had a bad day or a tough training session?" Invariably, every hand shoots up, and that's my opportunity to point out that those hard days are the ones where they likely learned the most.

Resiliency thrives on how we frame our experiences. A setback can either be a roadblock or a stepping stone, depending on how you choose to view it. When something doesn't work, the resilient person doesn't just get back up to repeat the same mistake. They adapt and find a new path. Rather than banging your head against a wall, they have the courage to bounce back, even if it means charting a completely new course.

Grit goes hand in hand with resilience, which is the ability to bounce back. Grit is the toughness that keeps you in the game when things get hard. As a wrestling coach, I saw grit develop in my athletes over time. When freshmen joined the team, many of them had no idea what it really took to become a state champion. They would tell me, "I want to be a state champ, Coach!" But they hadn't yet experienced the grueling training, the sacrifices, or the mental toughness required. At that stage, their "grit level" might be a one or two out of ten. Fortunately, grit isn't fixed—it can be built.

I think of grit like armor. At first, you might only have a small piece—a single armband. But with each practice, each challenge, you add another piece: a chest plate, another armband, a helmet. Over time, you're fully equipped to handle whatever life throws at you. That's the power of grit. It's the cumulative result of showing up day after day and refusing to quit.

SETTING THE TONE FOR THE DAY

We talked about this before, but it's so important that I want to tie it into resilience. You see, one of the simplest and most effective ways to practice resiliency and build momentum is by winning the morning. The morning sets the tone for the rest of your day, and creating small wins early on can have a compounding effect.

Winning the morning starts with small, intentional actions. Hydrate as soon as you wake up. Get some movement in, whether that's a short walk or a few stretches. Expose yourself to natural light or even blue light to align your circadian rhythms. These simple habits create a ripple effect that carries into the rest of your day.

For me, mornings are sacred. I like to combine movement with creativity and personal growth. I might knock out a simple task—nothing demanding, just enough to shift my energy—while a podcast plays in the background and my thoughts start to fall into place. Some mornings, I'll practice breathwork or meditation to center myself. Other days, I'll dive into a book or an audiobook to absorb new insights.

As we discussed earlier, nutrition is incredibly important. Whether I'm fasting or starting the day with a balanced meal, I make intentional choices to fuel my body and mind. None of this is overly complicated, but it works because it's consistent.

When I work with clients who struggle with mornings, we start small. If they're hitting snooze three times before rushing out the door, the first win is simply waking up thirty minutes earlier. That small adjustment might take a week or two to feel natural, but once it sticks, it creates momentum. Remember: *Movement creates motivation.*

Winning the morning doesn't mean you need a perfect routine from the get-go. Start with one or two actions, and let those wins build on each other. The key is to create habits that align with your goals and give you the best shot at owning the rest of your day.

Whether you're practicing resiliency, building grit, or focusing on winning the morning, it all comes down to small, consistent actions. Success isn't about huge leaps but tiny steps that add up over time. The beauty of this approach is that anyone can do it. You don't need to suddenly overhaul your whole life. You just need to take one step today and another tomorrow.

So, put on your armor, take a deep breath, and commit to dripping into the process. Small wins will carry you further than you ever thought possible. The journey won't always be easy, but if you stay the course, you'll discover just how capable you really are.

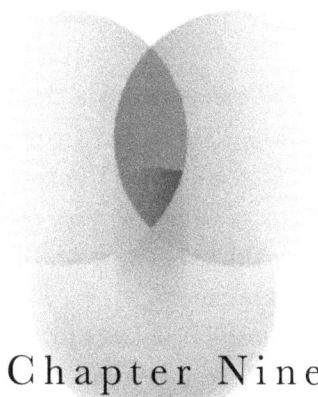

Chapter Nine

STAYING COMMITTED

COMMITMENT DOESN'T ALWAYS start with fireworks and a sprint toward the finish line. For many, it begins with barely a whisper of momentum. But if you can just get one or two small commitments rolling, they can snowball into something bigger. This idea is universal. High performers, whether they're in business, athletics, or the arts, rarely begin at the top of their game. Their journey often starts with small wins that build confidence and set the stage for larger achievements.

Take Tyler Hubbard, a wrestler I coached in high school. Tyler didn't walk into our wrestling room as a superstar. He'd placed sixth at the youth state tournament, but that's not exactly rare. Many kids eventually place at some level. What set Tyler apart wasn't natural talent but an unrelenting commitment to improvement. Tyler wrote down his goals and taped them to the ceiling above his bed. Every morning when he woke up and every night before he fell asleep, he would see those goals staring back at him. That was his level of commitment—total immersion.

It paid off. Tyler became a three-time state champion, winning his final title his senior year despite tearing his ACL during the tournament. He went on to win an NCAA Division III national championship at Wartburg College. His commitment evolved over time—from a kid with modest success in youth wrestling to a high school standout and eventually a collegiate champion.

What's remarkable about Tyler's story isn't just the hardware he earned but how his commitment grew with each stage of his journey. As his vision expanded, so did his dedication.

As a coach, I've learned that someone's commitment level today often has little bearing on where they'll be in two or five years. Momentum is a powerful thing. Once people experience small wins, their confidence grows, and so does their willingness to commit further.

Of course, some people are born with natural talent or access to incredible resources, and they might achieve a certain level of success without a ton of commitment. However, the real magic happens when someone pairs an unwavering commitment with consistent effort over time. That's when high performance becomes inevitable.

THE ROLE OF GOALS

When I developed the AOC model, I almost called it the AOA model because I felt that *action* was the heart of commitment. Ultimately, I went with AOC, but it's important to realize that the *C* in AOC doesn't just stand for commitment—it represents a *commitment to action*.

This is where the rubber meets the road. It's one thing to be aware of your situation and to take ownership of your role in it, but without action, those insights are meaningless. Commitment is what bridges the gap between intention and execution. This is where you lay out what you want to achieve and start taking deliberate steps toward it.

STAYING COMMITTED

Remember: it's not enough to write down your goals—you need to align your actions with those goals every single day.

You might start with a single, small commitment—like showing up to practice or getting out of bed thirty minutes earlier—but it's that initial action that sets everything else into motion. So, as you think about your own journey, ask yourself: What small commitment can I make today? It doesn't have to be monumental. In fact, it's better if it's not.

Don't worry about perfection. Instead, strive for consistency. Whether your long-term goal is to win a championship, launch a business, or improve your health, the formula remains the same: **Take action. Build momentum. Stay the course.** It all begins with that first small step.

Goals give us direction, but without a plan or timeline, they're just daydreams. I remember hearing a saying years ago: "Goals without a deadline are just dreams." That stuck with me, and for good reason. A goal is only as strong as the plan and timeframe behind it. Take, for example, the goal we set for our wrestling team at Blue Springs High School. We aimed to win the state championship within five years. As in the earlier example of us winning the team state wrestling tournament, we had set the goal, including a timeline of 5 years, which we came close to. Then, the very next year, we accomplished what we had set out to do. Without that clear timeline, the goal might have felt too abstract, too far off, or maybe even unattainable.

Again, when setting goals, I believe in aligning them with your vision and values. Goals that resonate deeply with your purpose are much easier to commit to. As a coach, I've heard countless goals from clients that sound great on the surface but lack genuine connection. People say what they think I want to hear—"I want to lose weight" or "I want to run a marathon"—but when we dig deeper, the *why* isn't strong enough to sustain the commitment.

For a goal to stick, it needs clarity. Vague resolutions like "I want to get healthier" are too easy to abandon. Instead, specificity and timeliness make all the difference: "I want to lose ten pounds in six months by walking ten thousand steps daily and eating more vegetables." Now we're talking!

In fact, there are *three* pillars of effective goal setting: clarity, consistency, and resiliency. Let's look at all three. To truly commit, you need these three essential elements working together.

The Pillars of Goal Setting

Clarity: A clear vision makes everything easier. If you know exactly where you're headed, you can plot the most effective course. It's like building a roadmap—you can't get to your destination if you don't know where it is. This is where goal setting intersects with the awareness phase we've talked about earlier.

So, why do so many people fail to pursue and achieve their goals? Think about New Year's resolutions. Most people who make bold resolutions on January 1 fail to follow through because their goals lack clarity and a strong why. They say things like, "I want to lose weight," but they don't specify how much or by when. And they often don't connect their goal to something meaningful.

Contrast that with someone whose doctor says, "If you don't lose twenty pounds in the next six months, your health will be at serious risk." That urgency provides clarity and a strong *why*, which makes commitment far more likely.

Consistency: If clarity is the map, consistency is the engine. Consistency isn't built in a week or a month; it's developed over years of steady action. Small, repeated efforts—what I've called "dripping into the process"—compound over time.

Remember: High performance isn't about grand gestures. It's about showing up every day, doing the work, and letting those daily actions stack up into something extraordinary. Consistency is what separates the dreamers from the doers.

Resiliency: As we've learned, this is your ability to bounce back when things go sideways—and they will. We've already discussed how setbacks are inevitable, but what defines a high performer is how they respond. If you can look at failures as learning opportunities instead of roadblocks, you're already ahead of the game.

Clarity, consistency, and resiliency combine to create the foundation of commitment. Without clarity, it's hard to stay consistent. Without consistency, you can't build resilience. And without resilience, even with clarity and consistency, one setback can derail your entire journey. These three work hand in hand.

Overcoming the Barriers to Commitment

While commitment is essential for success, there are several common barriers that can stop you in your tracks. Let's explore a few of these and how to address them.

Impatience: Impatience is a silent killer of commitment. We live in a world of instant gratification, but success often requires delayed rewards. Whether you're trying to lose weight, build a business, or master a skill, the results won't show up overnight.

Think about how growth actually happens—it's almost never linear. Progress often starts slow, with frustrating plateaus along the way. But if you stay patient, the fruits of your labor will come. As the old saying goes, patience is a virtue, and in the realm of commitment, it's nonnegotiable.

Burnout: Burnout often arises when there's no visible progress or when the process feels stagnant. From my experience coaching athletes and clients, burnout isn't just about working too hard; it's about working hard without seeing growth or learning something new.

Whether it's weight loss, improving athletic performance, improving relationships, or making progress in your career, if the results aren't there, it's easy to feel stuck. To combat burnout, focus on incremental progress. Even tiny improvements can reignite your motivation and keep the fire burning.

Fear of Discomfort: Discomfort is often the doorway to growth, but many people see it as a stop sign. High performers, however, recognize that being uncomfortable is a positive signal—it means you're being challenged.

When you feel uncomfortable, you can respond positively in one of two ways: push through and grow or pivot and learn. Either way, discomfort leads to progress. Instead of avoiding it, flip the script. See discomfort as a sign you're on the right path. It's a growth opportunity, not a threat.

So, how do you strengthen your commitment? Here's a practical approach:

1) **Break Your Goals into Manageable Steps.** One of the best ways to stay committed is to break your larger goals into smaller, actionable pieces. For example, instead of saying, "I want to lose fifty pounds," start with, "I'm going to drink more water and walk ten minutes a day." These smaller steps make the bigger goal feel less overwhelming and build momentum.

2) **Celebrate Small Wins.** Recognizing your progress, no matter how small, fuels your motivation, so celebrate each milestone, whether you're sticking to a workout routine for a week or hitting your first sales target. Small victories lead to big accomplishments.

3) **Reframe Discomfort.** Instead of fearing or trying to avoid discomfort, embrace it as a sign of growth. When you push through challenges—whether physical, mental, or

emotional—you build resilience. Growth rarely happens in your comfort zone, so learn to see discomfort as a friend, not a foe.
4) **Practice Patience.** Understand that real, lasting success takes time. Commit to the long game. Whether you're training for a marathon or launching a new business, patience will keep you grounded when results take longer than expected.
5) **Keep Learning.** When progress stalls, it's often because you've stopped learning. Seek out new techniques, fresh ideas, or updated strategies to keep things exciting. Growth comes from constant curiosity and a willingness to adapt.

Remember: Commitment is more than just sticking to a plan. It's about trusting the process, even when the results aren't immediately visible. Focus on what's doable right now, stay patient, and continue building. Progress isn't about diving in—it's about staying consistent.

TRACKING PROGRESS AND CELEBRATING WINS

A few weeks ago (at the time of this writing), I spoke to a group of coaches and was asked about the most important elements of building a successful program. I responded by talking about the importance of establishing routines and systems. These systems act as your guide rails, ensuring you stay on track day in and day out. They're not static either. Your routines need regular review and adjustment to keep you moving forward.

Tracking progress is equally important. Remember: Progress creates motivation (not the other way around). I've seen this firsthand in my own journey. When I started college wrestling, those first two or three months were *rough*. I was constantly getting beaten in the practice room—barely landing a takedown. I felt like

I was going backward, not forward, but during a holiday break, I returned to my high school and trained with younger wrestlers I used to struggle against. To my amazement, I dominated them. That experience made me realize how far I'd come. My measuring stick in the college room had been skewed, which hid the progress I was actually making.

Be mindful of how you measure success. Sometimes, we need to zoom out and reflect on how far we've come. Metrics matter, but they must be meaningful, realistic, and contextually appropriate.

As a high performer, it's easy to focus on the "what's-next" mentality. You hit one goal, and immediately, you're eyeing the next challenge. I've been guilty of this myself—winning a state title and, instead of savoring the moment, already planning the next season. The constant pursuit of *more* can blind you to the joy of the present.

Celebrate your wins, both big and small. It will keep you inspired and engaged. Just because you pause to celebrate doesn't mean you're abandoning ambition. On the contrary, you are appreciating the journey. Gratitude is a powerful tool, and pausing to acknowledge your progress creates a deeper sense of fulfillment. So, yes, plan for what's next—but don't forget to enjoy the victory lap.

Tools and Strategies

If you're serious about reaching your goals and staying committed, you need tools in your toolbox that help keep you on track. One of the most powerful tools I recommend is a *weekly action plan*. This is where your goals take shape in a tangible, manageable way. By planning your week around your key goals and tasks, you give your commitment structure. Progress is no longer abstract. Now, it's actionable.

Another tool I often recommend when coaching is *habit tracking*. When I start working with someone, I always ask them to track their habits for two weeks. I want to see what their day looks like from morning to night, broken into thirty-minute chunks. This is important because *habits define progress*. Once we uncover those patterns, we can tweak and optimize them. It's often eye-opening for people to realize how much time they're wasting—or how many hidden opportunities for growth they're missing.

Don't underestimate the importance of *accountability*. For years, I maintained an informal network of peers—coaches, officials, and mentors—to bounce ideas off of and get feedback. Today, I've leveled that up by working with a professional coach and participating in a mastermind group. Every two weeks, we meet to share wins, losses, and strategies. Whether it's through a professional coach, a mastermind group, or even just an accountability buddy, having someone to help keep you on track makes a huge difference. Don't view this as an expense—view it as an investment in yourself.

Energy management is another important piece of the puzzle. If you don't know when you're at your best—mentally, physically, and creatively—you're working against yourself. Take stock of your energy levels throughout the day.

For me, mornings are when I'm at my most creative. I do my best creative work from about 10:00 a.m. to noon. That's when my mind is sharpest and I'm most focused, so I block out time for writing or brainstorming. After that, like I said, I shift to more routine tasks like responding to emails or organizing my schedule. Strength training is in the afternoon when my energy is more suited for physical exertion.

Finding these peak times in your own day can help tremendously with consistency. You'll feel more productive and motivated to get things done when you're working *with*, not *against*, your natural energy cycles. By aligning your tasks with your natural rhythms, you optimize your performance and stay committed without feeling drained.

For that reason, I believe energy management is just as important as time management. People often think progress is all about working harder, but working *smarter* is what matters most. That means knowing when you're at your best and scheduling your most important tasks during those peak energy periods. For some, it's in the morning when creativity is at its highest. For others, it's later in the day.

An underrated tool is *visualization*. If you can see it in your mind, you're much more likely to make it happen. When I visualize, I don't picture failure; I only imagine success. I'm not talking about wishful thinking. Rather, this is about mentally rehearsing the steps you'll take to achieve your goals. Visualization builds confidence and helps you strategize. Whether I'm working on this book or thinking about my next big project, I spend time visualizing the path forward. It's like a mental dry run that makes the real thing feel that much more attainable.

Finally, you need to define your *personal mission statement*. This is your ultimate "why." What are you trying to accomplish in your life? What's your purpose? High performers have clarity on this—they know their core values and use them as a compass to guide their decisions and actions. Your mission statement isn't just a fancy phrase you jot down once; it's the guiding light for everything you achieve. When you pair it with tools like visualization and action plans, you create unstoppable momentum.

By breaking your goals into manageable chunks, setting up a system for accountability, and understanding when you work best, you set yourself up for sustainable success. Each of these tools is part of the process of committing to your growth. It's about creating the right environment for progress while staying aligned with your values and priorities.

STAYING COMMITTED

Tackling Challenges of Any Size

At its heart, the AOC model is a framework for tackling challenges of any size. It works just as well for solving specific problems as it does for reshaping your entire life. **Awareness** helps you understand where you are and what's around you. **Ownership** gives you the power to take charge. And **Commitment** is where you roll up your sleeves and get to work.

What I love most about this model is its flexibility. Whether you're focusing on a single challenge or a global transformation, AOC gives you the tools and mindset to move forward. It's a strategy you can apply to every aspect of your life, from parenting to career growth to personal development.

Don't wait for the perfect moment to start. Take control one step at a time. By aligning your energy, building accountability, and visualizing success, you create a system that drives progress and fosters growth. Whether you're tackling a small goal or reimagining your life, the AOC model is here to help you take that first step—and the next, and the next.

Part Five

BRINGING IT ALL TOGETHER

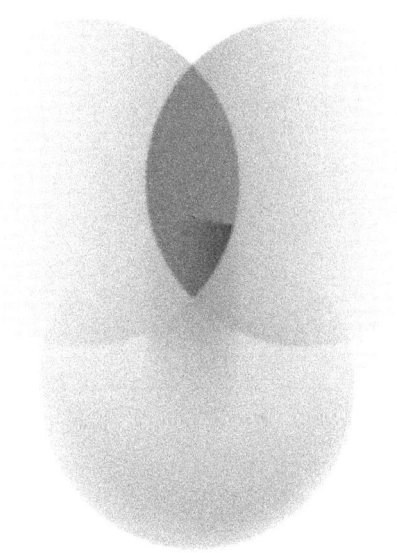

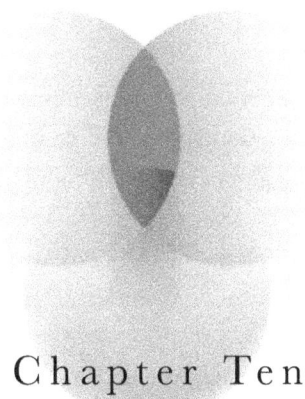

Chapter Ten

INTEGRATING AOC INTO DAILY LIFE

AWARENESS, OWNERSHIP, AND commitment. These three elements at the heart of the AOC model aren't just stand-alone ideas. They work together like gears in a well-oiled machine. If you lack **awareness**, you don't even know where to start. If you lack **ownership**, you'll always find excuses. And if you lack **commitment**, you'll never follow through. But when you put them together, that's when the magic happens. That's when transformation takes place.

Of course, no one is just one thing. You're not just a husband, just a wife, just an employee, just a business owner, or just a coach. You are a complex individual with many different roles, responsibilities, relationships, and priorities. High performance isn't about mastering only one aspect of your life—it's about showing up at your best in the areas that matter most to you. That's the key: High performance is a choice, and it's up to each person to decide where to apply it.

For me, high performance means excelling in my career, being a dedicated father and grandparent, and continuously growing as a coach. These are my biggest priorities. But for you, the equation may look entirely different. That's the beauty of it. There's no one-size-fits-all formula for success, which is why this book isn't about rigid steps or a prescriptive checklist. It's about a mindset. It's about understanding how to apply awareness, ownership, and commitment—the AOC model—to whatever aspect of your life you want to improve.

However, before you can take action, you have to be honest with yourself. And that starts with awareness.

APPLYING AWARENESS

As we mentioned earlier, most people *think* they are self-aware, However, studies suggest that only 10 to 15 percent of people actually are.[9] That means the vast majority of us are walking around with blind spots, not fully understanding our own skills, traits, or tendencies. We assume we see ourselves clearly, but more often than not, our self-perception is vastly different from how others see us.

Self-awareness isn't self-criticism or beating yourself up over your weaknesses. It's about stepping back and taking a real, honest inventory. Ask yourself: *What are my strengths? What areas do I need to improve? What patterns keep repeating in my life that I might not be fully recognizing?* These are tough questions, but they are necessary ones.

Some of this self-awareness comes from reflection—taking the time to pause, evaluate, and ask yourself where you are and where you want to be. But gathering hard data is just as important. Remember: Without awareness, there's no growth. You can't fix what you refuse to see.

---

9   Jeff Kauflin, "Only 15% of People Are Self-Aware—Here's How to Change," *Forbes*, May 10, 2017, https://www.forbes.com/sites/jeffkauflin/2017/05/10/only-15-of-people-are-self-aware-heres-how-to-change/.

Self-awareness is more than just understanding our strengths and weaknesses. It's about recognizing how we show up—not just for ourselves, but for others. Are we radiating positivity and confidence, or are we carrying stress and frustration like twin badges of honor? Are we adding value to conversations, or are we draining energy from the room?

Think about the people you love being around. They bring life, energy, and a sense of possibility, no matter the situation. Now think about the people who seem to suck the oxygen out of the room—always complaining, always negative, always focusing on what's wrong instead of what's possible.

Now, ask yourself: *Which one am I?*

How are we showing up in our relationships, in our work, and in our daily interactions? Are we actively contributing, or are we passively waiting for things to happen to us?

Personal Mantra

One of the most powerful tools in this respect is a *personal mantra*. This is a declaration of who you are striving to become. At first, it might feel like blind faith, but putting it into words gives it power.

My personal mantra is simple: *"I am a high performer who is blessed to share time with other high performers on this planet."*

This statement reminds me every day of the kind of person I want to be and the people I want to surround myself with. I want to be in the company of others who strive to be their best because one of the hardest things for me has always been working with people who don't want to put in the effort.

Think about your own mantra. What do you want to be known for? What kind of life do you want to lead? Whether it's about being the best parent you can be, excelling in your career, or committing to a healthier lifestyle, crafting a clear and intentional statement helps you stay on course.

THE ART OF LISTENING

A foundational skill that ties into every part of the AOC model—but *especially* awareness—is the ability to listen. True listening is one of the most overlooked yet powerful skills in achieving high performance.

At its core, communication is simple: A sender delivers a message, a receiver receives it, and ideally, there's a loop of feedback. However, in between, there's something that disrupts the process—*distortion*. Distortion happens when distractions, assumptions, biases, or emotions get in the way of truly understanding a message.

High performers listen with intent. They aren't just waiting for their turn to speak. They absorb, process, and respond thoughtfully. Listening builds stronger relationships, sharpens decision-making, and increases awareness—both of yourself and of the world around you. If you want to excel in any area of life, master the art of listening. It will make you a better leader, a better partner, and a better performer in every arena.

I've had the opportunity to give presentations on the power of listening, and what continues to amaze me is how much people *think* they are listening when, in reality, they are just waiting for their turn to talk. High performers know how to separate noise from value. They take in feedback, process it for what it is—*information*, not a personal attack—and use it accordingly.

Take losing a job as an example. Most people immediately internalize that as a failure. But what if it's just data? What if the company was downsizing? What if this was an opportunity to land an even better job? The moment we remove the emotional baggage from feedback, we can use it to our advantage.

This applies to all aspects of life—career, relationships, personal growth. When you start listening to what's being said (or what's not being said), you gain clarity. What are your peers and mentors saying? What patterns keep coming up in conversations? What feedback do you keep dismissing because it's uncomfortable? That discomfort might be exactly what you need to hear.

This is something I've noticed time and time again. The highest performers—the best athletes, the most successful leaders—are always the ones *asking the most questions*. They actively seek feedback, not because they doubt themselves, but because they know growth comes from learning.

Growing up, I didn't always appreciate the lessons that came my way. In third grade, I attended a tiny Catholic school—so small, in fact, that it had only *two rooms*. The "little room" housed first through fourth grade, and the "big room" covered fifth through eighth. One nun taught *all* the students in each room. Looking back, I can't even imagine how the nuns managed it, but they did.

I was young for my grade—a May baby—which put me at a slight disadvantage in terms of maturity and development. Years later, I came across Malcolm Gladwell's book *Outliers*, which explores how birthdates can significantly impact success, especially in competitive environments. The older kids, simply by being a few months ahead in development, often have an edge. I, on the other hand, was born late in the school year and naturally struggled to keep up with my peers.

Even so, that school taught me a lot—not just about academics, but about adaptability. I had to learn by observing. I had to listen because the lessons weren't always directed at me. It was there, in that tiny two-room school, that I first discovered that we can learn from anything if we pay attention and truly *listen*.

Ownership: You Are the Driver

John Gordon, in his book *The Energy Bus*, lays out a simple but profound truth: *You are the driver of your own bus*. In other words, no one else ultimately controls your journey. No one else determines your destination. This is at the heart of *ownership*. You can't delegate responsibility for your own success. You have control over how you respond to challenges, how you process setbacks, and how you move forward. And the moment you fully accept that responsibility, your life changes.

Too often, people blame external circumstances—the economy, their boss, bad luck—but the most successful people don't waste time blaming. They focus on what they can control. They take the wheel and drive.

If a relationship feels one-sided, are we truly investing in it, or are we expecting the other person to do all the heavy lifting? If work feels stagnant, are we showing up with energy and ideas, or are we waiting for someone else to motivate us?

Ownership isn't about guilt or self-criticism—it's about *empowerment*. When we own our impact, we take back control. Instead of reacting to life, we start designing it.

Complacency: The Enemy of High Performance

Most people spend their lives chasing convenience, ease, and familiarity. They are complacent and try to avoid discomfort, and in doing so, they unknowingly block their own potential. On the other hand, high performers *seek out* discomfort. Whether it's physical stress in the gym or mental strain in solving a tough problem, growth only happens when we push beyond what's easy. The body adapts under resistance—muscles grow when they're challenged. The mind works the same way.

If you never stretch yourself, you will never expand your capabilities. Complacency is the enemy of high performance. If you stay in a space where everything is predictable, where you never feel challenged, you aren't going to grow.

This is one of the biggest and most significant mindset shifts you can make if you want to become a high performer in any area of life.

Embrace discomfort as a sign that you're on the right path. Instead of resisting stress, lean into it. Instead of backing away from a difficult task, see it as proof that you're pushing forward. This applies to everything—stepping into leadership roles, taking on new challenges, learning new skills. The people who truly succeed are the ones who intentionally put themselves in situations where they must adapt and evolve.

This is one of the biggest challenges I see when working with clients, whether in business, athletics, or personal development. They resist discomfort and challenges. They want to grow, they want to improve, but they struggle with the uncomfortable realities that come with change.

Take something as simple as getting up thirty minutes earlier to win the morning. It sounds easy enough, but the moment that alarm clock goes off, discomfort kicks in. Hitting snooze becomes almost instinctive. Or consider someone trying to level up in their career but hesitating to have a tough conversation with their boss or spouse about expectations. Change is uncomfortable. Growth is uncomfortable. But what feels uncomfortable today can become routine tomorrow.

The key is to find *manageable* ways to challenge yourself—not to take on overwhelming obstacles that leave you feeling defeated, but to seek out small wins that create progress. The goal isn't to push yourself to the brink of burnout. Again, it's to build *momentum*. And momentum, once it starts, is powerful.

The hardest part of any journey is getting started. It takes effort to push the boulder into motion, but once it's rolling, it doesn't take much to keep it going. This is why I focus so much on finding small victories for my clients—because success, no matter how small, fuels motivation and reinforces belief in what's possible.

Success isn't about waiting for the right conditions. It's about taking ownership, listening with intent, and actively choosing the path of growth—even when it's uncomfortable.

- **Listen to feedback**—not just what you want to hear, but what you *need* to hear.
- **Own your journey**—no one else is driving your bus.
- **Seek discomfort**—because that's where real transformation happens.

The road to high performance isn't smooth, and it's not supposed to be. The more you embrace that reality, the more unstoppable you become.

COMMITMENT AND THE LONG GAME

As we've said, the journey to high performance isn't about quick fixes or overnight transformations. It's about long-term commitment. I've worked with many athletes, professionals, and business owners over the years, and the biggest difference between those who succeed and those who don't succeed isn't talent or resources. It's commitment. It's the willingness to stay in the game, even when progress is slow and even when obstacles arise.

The key to commitment is *momentum*. You don't have to go full speed from day one. In fact, most high performers don't. They focus on one or two priorities, gain traction, and then expand from there. The mistake most people make is thinking they need to have everything figured out before they start. They wait for motivation, for the "perfect time." But momentum isn't built by waiting—it's built by *moving*—through consistent, intentional action. That's the difference. That's what commitment looks like.

So, as you move forward, ask yourself the following:
- *Where do I want to be a high performer?*
- *What blind spots do I need to address?*
- *What mantra will keep me focused and motivated?*

- *Am I truly listening—to myself, to others, to the lessons life is teaching me?*
- *Am I committed to taking consistent action, even when it's hard?*

By answering these questions and applying the AOC framework, you'll create lasting, meaningful change in whatever area of life matters most to you. Start making progress one step at a time, one win at a time, one commitment at a time.

Commitment Is a Lifestyle

Being a high performer isn't about having one great day. It's a lifestyle choice. It's not something you turn on when it's convenient and shut off when you're tired. It's a commitment to consistently operating at your best in the areas that matter most to you. High performance is built on decisions. Every day, you make choices about what to focus on, where to invest your time, how to respond to setbacks, and those choices determine your trajectory. Some people choose to coast and stay within their comfort zone. Others choose to lean into the work that leads to growth.

I'm not suggesting that you need to be hustling every moment of the day or be "excellent" 24/7. Rather, it's about identifying your priorities, whether that's your career, your health, your relationships, or something else, and showing up fully in those areas.

Once you set a goal, obstacles will appear. They always do. That's why it's so important to anticipate them. If you've tried to reach a goal before and didn't succeed, what got in your way? Was it a lack of time? A lack of support? A fear of failure? The problem is rarely the goal itself—it's how we handle resistance when it shows up. High performers don't see obstacles as stop signs. They see them as problems to solve, workarounds to find, or challenges to push through.

Every self-help book out there has some version of the resiliency story—the entrepreneur who failed multiple times before succeeding, the athlete who faced endless setbacks before winning, the leader who struggled before thriving. But *those stories aren't exceptions.* They are the rule for anyone pursuing high performance.

If you let the first roadblock derail you, you weren't fully committed in the first place. Real commitment means adapting, learning, and continuing forward no matter what. One of the biggest lessons I've learned from working with high performers is their ability to stay present while still keeping a vision for the future. They don't dwell on past failures. They don't obsess over distant outcomes. They focus on what they can do today to move forward.

This is a mindset shift that makes all the difference. Instead of thinking, *I failed before, so I'll probably fail again*, high performers think, *That was then. This is now. What's my next best step?*

They have a long-term vision, yes, but they don't let that vision overwhelm them. They take it one action at a time, trusting that small, consistent efforts will lead to big results.

So, if you're serious about becoming a high performer, embrace discomfort. Not in a way that crushes you but in a way that challenges you to stretch beyond where you are now.

- Find small wins to build momentum.
- Choose high performance as a lifestyle, not a one-time act.
- Take inventory of where you are today so you can make intentional changes.
- Expect obstacles—and plan your response before they show up.
- Stay present, focus on what you can control, and take it one step at a time.

High performance doesn't mean becoming perfect. It just means you are fully committed, and that's a choice you can make every single day.

Working Smarter

For years, I operated under the idea that grinding nonstop was the key to success. Work, work, work, with very little reflection—that was how I tried to live. While that approach certainly kept me busy, it didn't always keep me effective. I was making some progress, but not necessarily in the most efficient or healthy way.

Gaining clarity changed everything, but I didn't truly begin to find clarity until I started incorporating breathwork and meditation into my routine. I was always moving too fast, always thinking about the next big thing. Slowing down felt counterintuitive, but I soon realized that when I shifted out of that fight-or-flight mode and into a more balanced state, I could actually see things more clearly. The big picture came into focus. I could reassess my priorities and make better decisions, so I wasn't just working hard but working in a way that truly aligned with my goals.

Clarity isn't something that happens by accident—it's something you make time for. Whether it's ten minutes a day or a structured reflection every weekend, taking that pause to recalibrate is incredibly important. It allows us to step back, adjust where needed, and move forward with confidence.

What You Can Control

One of the biggest challenges in both high performance and personal growth is recognizing what you actually have control over. We all want certain things for our kids, our spouses, and our careers, but not everything is within our power. The key is to take inventory and ask, "What do I really control?"

You *can't* control other people's actions or external circumstances, but you *can* control your effort, your attitude, and your commitment to showing up. And showing up is half the battle.

One of my professors at Central Missouri used to say, "Anytime you attend a lecture, a meeting, or even have a conversation, make sure you walk away with at least one valuable takeaway." That advice stuck with me. Ever since, I've tried to approach every situation as a learning opportunity. That doesn't just apply to formal education or professional development. It applies to everything—whether it's a podcast I listen to on a morning walk, a conversation with a stranger, or even watching how someone else handles a frustrating situation. Every moment holds the potential for a lesson, but only if you're paying attention.

I was always a restless kid, full of energy, and honestly, school frustrated me. I remember vividly walking home one afternoon, carrying my books and papers, feeling utterly defeated by my subpar academic performance. As I passed by an incinerator, where people used to openly burn trash, I stopped, stared at the fire, and, without hesitation, tossed everything I was carrying into the flames. Watching those books burn felt liberating. I hated school. I didn't see the point of learning.

Unfortunately, my moment of rebellion didn't go unnoticed. A nun happened to be standing on the back porch of the school, watching the whole thing unfold. Let's just say my parents weren't exactly thrilled when they found out. But at that time in my life, I was stuck. I felt behind. I was one of the youngest in my grade, surrounded by kids who were born months earlier and who seemed just a little more physically and mentally developed than I was. It took me years before I realized that my struggles weren't a reflection of my intelligence—they were a reflection of my mindset.

Things started to shift in high school when I discovered wrestling. For the first time, I saw purpose in working hard, and I started to understand how education fits into the bigger picture since I couldn't wrestle if I didn't keep my grades up. That realization was a turning point. Suddenly, school wasn't just something I had to endure. It became a tool that allowed me to do what I loved.

That experience showed me that people don't always start at the same place. Everyone comes into their personal growth journey at a different level of awareness, ownership, and commitment. Some people are ready to go all in, fueled by a major life event or a rock-bottom moment. Others need time to warm up to the idea of change, testing the waters before diving in. And that's OK. The important thing is that you start—wherever that may be.

COMMITMENT STARTS WITH ACTION

One of the biggest myths about commitment is that you have to feel ready before you begin. The truth, as we've said, is that action comes first.

I was working with a client recently who had struggled with consistency for years. She told me, "I finally understand what you mean about movement creating motivation." She had spent so much of her life waiting to feel inspired before taking action. When she was in the mood, she performed at a high level. But when she wasn't, she stalled out completely. Now, she's flipped the script. On days she doesn't feel like doing anything, she forces herself to put on her shoes and go for a walk. That small action often snowballs into something bigger. Some days, she keeps walking. Other days, she heads to the gym. But no matter what, she moves—and that movement creates momentum.

To help you get moving, I recommend using a *schedule* where you carve out specific time for activities. To-do lists are great, but if you don't make time on your calendar for the things that matter, they often get pushed aside. I put everything important on my Google Calendar—not just meetings or deadlines, but workouts, self-reflection time, and even new routines I want to try.

I don't just schedule events. I also add descriptions to them. If I plan a workout, I'll drop in the details—what exercises I'm doing, the focus for that session. When I was coaching wrestling, I used to create my practice plans in my calendar so my team and fellow coaches could see them in advance. It kept everyone on the same page.

Life gets busy. Other priorities will try to take over, but if something is on your calendar, it becomes real. You're making a commitment to yourself, and that commitment, repeated over time, is what separates those who achieve their goals from those who simply dream about them.

BECOMING BETTER SO WE CAN GIVE MORE

The beauty of the AOC model is that it's not just about *us*—it's about making ourselves better so we can be better for the people around us.

Some people might look at self-improvement as selfish, but that's the furthest thing from the truth. When we grow, when we take ownership of our lives, and when we show up with energy and purpose, we become the type of people who inspire, support, and elevate those around us.

That's the real goal. Not just personal success but personal impact.

So ask yourself: *How am I showing up today? And how can I make sure I show up better tomorrow?*

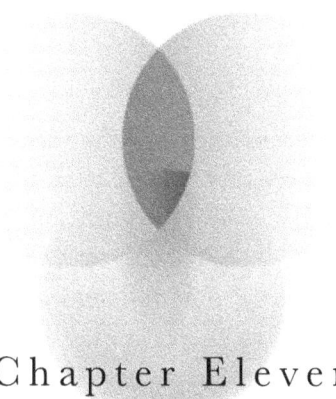

Chapter Eleven

SUSTAINING HIGH PERFORMANCE

TOO OFTEN, WHEN people embark on a self-improvement journey, they overwhelm themselves with massive expectations. They try to change everything at once, set unrealistic goals, and then feel discouraged when they don't immediately see results. That's not how sustainable growth works. The real secret is to start with one simple, achievable thing.

When I work with clients, whether in high performance coaching or health coaching, I always ask, "What do you want to focus on first? What's the one area in your life where making a small but meaningful improvement would create a ripple effect?" Once that first challenge is tackled successfully, it builds confidence. That small win creates momentum, and suddenly, the next challenge doesn't seem so overwhelming.

There's nothing more fulfilling than watching someone accomplish a goal and share their excitement. As a coach, when I hear someone say, "Hey, you know what? I did that thing we talked about, and it actually worked!"—that's the highlight of my day. Because I know that once they've seen success, they're going to trust the process. They'll trust *themselves*. And that trust is what fuels long-term commitment.

High performance isn't something you *achieve* like a trophy you put on the shelf. There's no finish line. You don't wake up one day and declare, "I'm officially a high performer. My work here is done."

High performers never stop improving. They are in a constant state of growth, reflecting on where they've been, assessing where they are, and identifying where they want to go next. That's the mindset of high performance. *You're not striving to reach a destination. You are committing to a new way of life.*

If someone evaluates themselves today and realizes they're not yet living as a high performer, that doesn't mean they can't get there. And if they do reach that level, it's not about maintaining it for a short time—it's about embedding those habits and mindsets into everyday life.

Ultimately, high performance means developing the resilience to overcome obstacles, the discipline to stay committed, and the self-awareness to know when adjustments are needed. It means having the adaptability to shift gears when life throws a curveball and the humility to recognize that there's always room to improve.

SELF-CARE IS NONNEGOTIABLE

This is where the conversation comes full circle. As we said in the beginning, you *cannot* sustain high performance without prioritizing self-care. I don't care how driven, ambitious, or talented someone is—if they neglect their physical and mental well-being, they will eventually burn out. Period.

Remember the four pillars of self-care that every high performer must integrate into their routine:

1. **Movement and Exercise**—a strong body supports a strong mind.
2. **Nutrition and Hydration**—what you put into your body affects your energy, clarity, and longevity.
3. **Sleep and Recovery**—prioritizing rest isn't lazy—it's a performance strategy.
4. **Stress Management and Mental Clarity**—whether through meditation, breathwork, or simply taking time for stillness, high performers make time to reset and recalibrate.

High performance and self-care are inseparable. If you want to operate at your highest level but you completely ignore your well-being, it's like trying to drive a high performance sports car with no oil in the engine. It won't last.

Just Start Somewhere

One of the most common things I hear from people when they first start this journey is, "I don't even know where to begin." That's completely normal. Everyone starts at a different place. There is no universal roadmap and no one-size fits-all formula.

Some people have a strong foundation but need small tweaks to optimize their performance. Others feel like they're starting from zero, overwhelmed by the idea of change. *It doesn't matter where you start. It only matters that you start.*

Ironically, those who feel they have the *least* to work with often experience the most dramatic growth. Small changes compound over time, and before they know it, they're operating at a level they never thought possible.

There's a reason why personal development books fly off the shelves, why people chase the next big "life hack" or productivity tool. But there are no shortcuts. Yes, strategies help. Yes, tools like wearables, trackers, and journals can be useful, but there is no replacement for consistently showing up and doing the work.

That's why action must always come before motivation. Too many people wait for inspiration to strike before they take action, but real high performers know that motivation follows movement.

The Power of Showing Up

At the end of the day, success—whether in business, fitness, relationships, or personal growth—boils down to one simple principle: Just show up.

Years ago, one of my college professors said something that stuck with me: "If you just show up, you're already ahead of half the people out there."

Think about it—how many people talk about wanting to improve but never take the first step? How many people set goals but quit at the first sign of difficulty? High performers *show up*, even when they don't feel like it. They don't wait for the perfect conditions, the perfect plan, the perfect timing, or the perfect day. They take action *now*, adjust along the way, and keep moving forward.

So, if there's one takeaway from all of this, it's this:
Start small. Take action. Build momentum. Prioritize self-care. Keep showing up.

Because high performance isn't a destination. It's a way of life.

CONCLUSION

AS I'VE SAID before (and it's worth saying again), success is not the destination. It's the journey. High performance is about embracing every step, every challenge, and every opportunity to grow. True progress doesn't come from waiting until everything is perfect; it comes from showing up, doing the work, and making the decision to move forward every single day.

One of the most powerful changes we can make is learning to express gratitude not just for the wins but for the hardships. That's where the real growth happens. It's in the struggles and the moments of uncertainty that we discover what we're truly capable of. But without awareness, ownership, and commitment—the elements of the AOC model— you won't get very far. These principles aren't just abstract concepts but the keys to unlocking your potential in every area of life.

So, where do you go from here? Start where you are. Right now. Today. Work on yourself. High performance isn't about making seven figures or having a perfect body—it's about being the best version of yourself in whatever you choose to pursue. It's about striving, growing, and refusing to settle for mediocrity.

And once you've made that commitment in your own life, the next step is sharing it. Help others rise. Surround yourself with people who challenge and inspire you—people who, like you, are committed to becoming better. Find partners, mentors, and a community that fuels your growth. There's a special kind of energy in those circles, an unstoppable momentum that comes from being around others who believe in continuous growth.

I recently attended a gathering of high performers in Kansas City—practitioners, coaches, counselors, and fitness experts—people from all walks of life, all committed to growth, both personally and in service to others. What stood out wasn't just their expertise but their mindset. They weren't fixated on limitations or obstacles. They were focused on possibilities. That's the kind of community that fuels transformation, and that's the kind of energy I want for you.

As you move forward, seek out the spaces, relationships, and resources that expand your thinking and push you to be more. Engage with communities that uplift and challenge you. Become part of a movement where growth isn't just personal but shared. Because the real magic happens not just in what you achieve, but in what you help others achieve along the way.

So here's your call to action: Step into your potential. Commit to the journey. Find your people. And never stop growing.

Let's build something extraordinary—together.

RESOURCES

Fifty Habits and Behaviors of High Performers

1. **Winning the Mornings**: High performers start their day with intention, often having a morning routine that includes exercise, meditation, or planning to set a positive tone for the day.
2. **Setting Clear Goals**: They establish specific, measurable, achievable, relevant, and time-bound (SMART) goals to focus their efforts and track progress.
3. **Prioritizing Health and Wellness**: They prioritize physical and mental health through regular exercise, a balanced diet, and adequate sleep.
4. **Continuous Learning**: High performers are lifelong learners, constantly seeking knowledge and skills to improve themselves and stay ahead.
5. **Practicing Gratitude**: They regularly acknowledge and appreciate the positive aspects of their lives, fostering a positive mindset.

6. **Effective Time Management**: They manage their time efficiently by scheduling tasks, avoiding procrastination, and focusing on high-impact activities.
7. **Maintaining a Growth Mindset**: They view challenges as opportunities to learn and grow rather than as threats.
8. **Developing Emotional Intelligence**: They are aware of and manage their emotions, and they empathize with others, building strong relationships.
9. **Staying Organized**: They keep their physical and digital spaces tidy, making it easier to focus and stay productive.
10. **Seeking Feedback and Reflecting**: They actively seek constructive feedback and reflect on their experiences to continuously improve.

Additional High performance Habits

11. **Networking and Building Relationships**: They invest time in building and maintaining professional and personal connections.
12. **Being Decisive**: They make decisions promptly and confidently, minimizing indecision and overthinking.
13. **Taking Ownership and Responsibility**: They take responsibility for their actions and outcomes, both successes and failures.
14. **Focusing on Solutions, Not Problems**: They concentrate on finding solutions rather than dwelling on obstacles.
15. **Maintaining a Positive Attitude**: They keep a positive attitude, even in the face of adversity, which helps them persevere.
16. **Staying Present and Mindful**: They practice mindfulness and stay present in the moment, reducing stress and enhancing focus. (I confess, *this one is difficult for me!*)
17. **Regularly Reviewing Progress**: They frequently assess their progress toward goals and adjust their strategies as needed.

18. **Being Adaptable and Resilient**: They adapt to changes and bounce back from setbacks quickly.
19. **Investing in Personal Development**: They regularly engage in personal development activities, such as reading books, attending seminars, or taking courses.
20. **Being Disciplined**: They maintain discipline in their actions, sticking to routines and plans even when it's challenging.
21. **Setting Boundaries**: They set clear boundaries to protect their time and energy.
22. **Engaging in Creative Outlets**: They explore creative activities to stimulate their minds and relieve stress.
23. **Being Charitable and Giving Back**: They give back to their communities and support causes they care about.
24. **Practicing Effective Communication**: They communicate clearly and effectively, both in speaking and writing.
25. **Taking Breaks and Practicing Self-Care**: They understand the importance of rest and regularly take breaks to recharge.
26. **Fostering a Supportive Environment**: They surround themselves with positive and supportive people.
27. **Leveraging Technology Wisely**: They use technology to enhance productivity without letting it become a distraction.
28. **Maintaining a Balanced Lif**e: They strive for a healthy work-life balance, making time for family, hobbies, and relaxation.
29. **Staying Curious**: They maintain a curious mindset, always asking questions and exploring new ideas.
30. **Being Persistent**: They persistently pursue their goals, even when faced with challenges or setbacks.
31. **Staying Informed**: They stay informed about current events and trends in their field and beyond.
32. **Cultivating Patience**: They practice patience, understanding that significant achievements often take time.

33. **Managing Finances Wisely**: They manage their finances responsibly, budgeting, saving, and investing prudently.
34. **Delegating Effectively**: They delegate tasks when appropriate, trusting others to help them achieve their goals.
35. **Seeking Mentors and Role Models**: They seek guidance and inspiration from mentors and role models.
36. **Embracing Diversity and Inclusivity**: They value diversity and inclusivity, fostering an environment of respect and understanding.
37. **Practicing Humility**: They remain humble and open to learning from others, regardless of their status or expertise.
38. **Maintaining a Sense of Humor**: They maintain a sense of humor, which helps them cope with stress and maintain perspective.
39. **Being Proactive**: They take initiative and act proactively rather than waiting for things to happen.
40. **Keeping a Journal**: They keep a journal to document thoughts, reflections, and progress.
41. **Celebrating Small Wins**: They celebrate small achievements along the way to stay motivated.
42. **Practicing Mindfulness Meditation**: They incorporate mindfulness meditation into their routine for mental clarity and stress reduction.
43. **Learning from Failure**: They view failure as a learning opportunity and extract valuable lessons from setbacks.
44. **Nurturing Creativity**: They engage in activities that nurture their creativity, such as art, music, or writing.
45. **Remaining Accountable**: They hold themselves accountable for their actions and commitments.
46. **Prioritizing Long-Term Success**: They focus on long-term success rather than short-term gains.

47. **Engaging in Regular Reflection**: They regularly reflect on their experiences and insights to grow personally and professionally.
48. **Building Strong Work Ethics**: They maintain a strong work ethic, demonstrating dedication and integrity in all they do.
49. **Embracing Challenges**: They embrace challenges and view them as opportunities for growth.
50. **Maintaining a Vision**: They have a clear vision of their future and work consistently toward realizing it.

Awareness, Ownership, Commitment (AOC) Model Assessment Tool

This assessment tool is designed to help individuals gauge their levels of awareness, ownership, and commitment. Each section contains fifteen questions, with five additional general questions to reflect overall alignment with the AOC model. Rate yourself on a scale of 1 to 5 for each statement, where:

1 = Strongly Disagree 2 = Disagree 3 = Neutral 4 = Agree 5 = Strongly Agree

Awareness

1. I clearly understand my strengths and weaknesses.
2. I regularly reflect on my personal and professional goals.
3. I am aware of how my emotions influence my decisions.
4. I recognize when I need to seek help or guidance.
5. I can identify patterns in my behavior that hold me back.
6. I am conscious of how my actions impact others.
7. I know what motivates me to perform at my best.

8. I frequently assess my progress toward achieving my goals.
9. I can adapt my plans based on new information or challenges.
10. I recognize when I am in a fixed mindset versus a growth mindset.
11. I am aware of how my environment affects my productivity.
12. I understand the connection between my physical and mental health.
13. I am aware of what I need to change to improve my life.
14. I actively seek feedback from others to improve.
15. I understand how my values influence my decisions.

Ownership

1. I take full responsibility for my successes and failures.
2. I follow through on the commitments I make to myself.
3. I am proactive in solving problems rather than waiting for others to act.
4. I own my role in conflicts and work to resolve them constructively.
5. I regularly evaluate how my habits affect my performance.
6. I take ownership of my time and prioritize effectively.
7. I hold myself accountable to the goals I set.
8. I am willing to do the hard work necessary to achieve my objectives.
9. I avoid making excuses for missed opportunities.
10. I embrace challenges as opportunities for growth.
11. I take ownership of my learning and seek resources to grow.
12. I actively work to improve my weaknesses.
13. I communicate openly about my needs and goals.
14. I am consistent in my actions, even when motivation is low.

15. I take initiative without being asked.

Commitment

1. I set clear and realistic goals for myself.
2. I break larger goals into smaller, manageable steps.
3. I maintain focus on my priorities despite distractions.
4. I stay committed to my goals, even when progress is slow.
5. I regularly review and adjust my goals as needed.
6. I embrace discipline as a key part of success.
7. I consistently show up for myself, even when it's inconvenient.
8. I put in extra effort when needed to reach my goals.
9. I maintain a positive attitude toward long-term efforts.
10. I set boundaries to protect my time and energy.
11. I celebrate small victories to stay motivated.
12. I track my progress to stay on course.
13. I prioritize my commitments over temporary comforts.
14. I seek accountability partners to stay consistent.
15. I remain resilient in the face of setbacks.

General Alignment with AOC

I feel balanced in my levels of awareness, ownership, and commitment.

I actively work to integrate awareness, ownership, and commitment into my daily life.

I can clearly identify how each area of the AOC model affects my success.

I am consistent in applying the principles of the AOC model.

I recognize the interconnectedness of awareness, ownership, and commitment.

Scoring

Step 1: Add up your scores for each section:
- Awareness: _____ / 75
- Ownership: _____ / 75
- Commitment: _____ / 75
- General alignment: _____ / 25

Step 2: Calculate your total score: _____ / 250

Step 3: Reflect on your scores:
- **200–250:** You are highly aligned with the AOC model and demonstrate strong high performance tendencies.
- **150–199:** You show good alignment but may have areas to develop further.
- **100–149:** There is room for significant growth in integrating awareness, ownership, and commitment into your life.
- **Below 100:** Focus on building the foundational elements of the AOC model in all areas.

Using Your Results
- Identify your highest and lowest sections. Where are you excelling? Where do you need to improve?
- Use your scores to create an action plan for strengthening your awareness, ownership, or commitment.
- Repeat this assessment every six months to track your growth and refine your high performance journey.

RECOMMENDED READING LIST

I'VE PUT TOGETHER a list of other books that can help you as you begin to make the elements of the AOC model part of your everyday routine. These are books that have helped me and others to achieve high performance in every area of life.

- *Own the Day, Own Your Life: Optimized Practices for Waking, Working, Learning, Eating, Training, Playing, Sleeping, and Sex* by Aubrey Marcus
- *Amplify Your Influence: Transform How You Communicate and Lead* by Rene Rodriguez
- *Buy Back Your Time: Get Unstuck, Reclaim Your Freedom, and Build Your Empire* by Dan Martell
- *Good Energy: The Surprising Connection Between Metabolism and Limitless Health* by Casey Means, MD
- *The Fitness Mindset: Eat for Energy, Train for Tension, Manage Your Mindset, Reap the Results* by Brian Keane
- *The School of Greatness: A Real-World Guide to Living Bigger, Loving Deeper, and Leaving a Legacy* by Lewis Howes

- *The Greatness Mindset: Unlock the Power of Your Mind and Live Your Best Life Today* by Lewis Howes
- *Outlive: The Science and Art of Longevity* by Peter Attia, MD
- *Mind Your Mindset: The Science That Shows Success Starts with Your Thinking* by Michael Hyatt, Megan Hyatt Miller
- *Sustain Your Game: High Performance Keys to Manage Stress, Avoid Stagnation, and Beat Burnout* by Alan Stein, Jon Sternfeld, Rece Davis
- *Beyond Grit: Ten Powerful Practices to Gain the High performance Edge* by Cindra Kamphoff
- *Master Mentors: 30 Transformative Insights from Our Greatest Minds* by Scott Jeffrey Miller
- *Your Pristine Blueprint: The Missing Key to Longevity, Reversing Disease, and Radically Transforming Your Life* by Beth McDougall, MD
- *Life Force: How New Breakthroughs in Precision Medicine Can Transform the Quality of Your Life & Those You Love* by Tony Robbins, Peter H. Diamandis, Robert Hariri
- *The Energy Formula: Six Life Changing Ingredients to Unleash Your Limitless Potential* by Shawn Wells, MPH RD LDN FISSN
- *Indistractable: How to Control Your Attention and Choose Your Life* by Nir Eyal, Julie Li
- *The Genius Life: Heal Your Mind, Strengthen Your Body, and Become Extraordinary (Genius Living, Book 2)* by Max Lugavere
- *Tools of Titans: The Tactics, Routines, and Habits of Billionaires, Icons, and World-Class Performers* by Tim Ferriss
- *Limitless: Upgrade Your Brain, Learn Anything Faster, and Unlock Your Exceptional Life* by Jim Kwik
- *Boundless: Upgrade Your Brain, Optimize Your Body & Defy Aging* by Ben Greenfield

- *Super Brain: Unleashing the Explosive Power of Your Mind to Maximize Health, Happiness, and Spiritual Well-Being* by Rudolph E. Tanzi, Deepak Chopra
- *The Fatburn Fix: Boost Energy, End Hunger, and Lose Weight by Using Body Fat for Fuel* by Catherine Shanahan, MD
- *Stress Less, Accomplish More: Meditation for Extraordinary Performance* by Emily Fletcher
- *Mastery* by Robert Greene
- *Atomic Habits: An Easy & Proven Way to Build Good Habits & Break Bad Ones* by James Clear
- *Claim Your Power* by Mastin Kipp
- *Willpower Doesn't Work* by Benjamin Hardy
- *How Successful People Think: Change Your Thinking, Change Your Life* by John C. Maxwell
- *Brain Rules: 12 Principles for Surviving and Thriving at Work, Home, and School* by John J. Medina
- *The Champion's Mind: How Great Athletes Think, Train, and Thrive* by Jim Afremow
- *The Subtle Art of Not Giving a F*ck: A Counterintuitive Approach to Living a Good Life* by Mark Manson
- *Grit: The Power of Passion and Perseverance* by Angela Duckworth
- *The Motivation Manifesto* by Brendon Burchard
- *The Miracle Morning: The Not-So-Obvious Secret Guaranteed to Transform Your Life (Before 8AM)* by Hal Elrod
- *High Performance Habits: How Extraordinary People Become That Way* by Brendon Burchard
- *The Energy Bus: 10 Rules to Fuel Your Life, Work, and Team with Positive Energy* by Jon Gordon

ACKNOWLEDGMENTS

FIRST AND FOREMOST, I want to thank my family, who have supported me throughout my journey as a teacher, coach, and NCAA wrestling official. To my wife, **Francesca**—your love and patience have been my foundation. To my son, **Keenan**, who endured having a dad as a coach for so many years—I know it wasn't always easy, but I hope you know how proud I am of you. To my daughters, **Michaela**, **Haley**, and **Mariah**—I appreciate your understanding through the many missed birthdays, events, and moments that come with having a father so deeply committed to his profession. Your love and support have meant everything to me.

To my parents, **John** and **Corky Hagerty**—thank you for instilling in me the values of hard work, integrity, and perseverance. Your love and guidance shaped the person I am today, and I am forever grateful.

To my high school coach, **Jim Cooper**—the "nutty professor" who lit a fire under a kid who had little direction before your influence. You saw something in me before I saw it in myself, and I will always be grateful for your passion and belief in me.

To my college coach, **Roger Denker**—thank you for taking a chance on a kid from the small town of Higginsville. The opportunity you gave me turned out to be one of the greatest blessings of my life. Your guidance extended far beyond the wrestling mat, shaping the path that led me here.

To my assistant coaches, both at the high school and college levels—your dedication and hard work made a lasting impact on countless student-athletes, and I am grateful for the opportunity to have worked alongside you. A special thank you to **Matt Cox** and **Jay Greco**, who not only helped hundreds of young athletes but also helped me grow as a coach and leader.

To the athletes I had the privilege of coaching at the high school, collegiate, and international levels—you have been my inspiration. Coaching you has been one of the greatest honors of my life.

To my teaching, coaching, and officiating peers—your dedication and passion have challenged me, shaped me, and made me a better teacher, coach, and official. I have learned so much from you, and I am grateful for the countless conversations, lessons, and experiences we have shared.

To my college teammates, who taught me invaluable lessons both on and off the mat—**Les Gatrel**, **Greg Anderson**, **Dave Streibig**, and **Jimmy May**—thank you for shaping me not just as an athlete but as a person. I learned so much from you, including humility and perseverance.

To **Gary Mayabb**, the brother I never had—through all our years of this lifelong adventure, in both coaching and officiating, your unwavering support and motivation continue to push me to be the best version of myself. Your influence has left a lasting mark on my life, and for that, I am forever grateful.

To my personal coaching clients, thank you for trusting me to be part of your journey. Your dedication to growth and high performance is inspiring, and working with you has been a privilege.

This book is dedicated to all of you.

ABOUT THE AUTHOR

MIKE HAGERTY'S JOURNEY in wrestling began as a competitor at Central Missouri State University, where he was an MIAA Champion and NCAA national qualifier. Transitioning into coaching, he led the University of Central Missouri's wrestling program for seven seasons. Under his guidance, the team produced two national champions, ten All-Americans, and twenty-five national qualifiers. He earned the Midwest Regional Coach of the Year title twice.

Hagerty's impact later extended to Blue Springs High School, where he served as head wrestling coach. His tenure was marked by three state championships and seven additional top-three finishes. He was honored as Missouri Coach of the Year five times and inducted into both the Missouri USA Wrestling Hall of Fame and the Missouri Wrestling Association Hall of Fame.

Beyond coaching, he has been a prominent NCAA Division I official for over twenty-five years, officiating numerous national championships and earning recognition as one of the nation's top collegiate referees. In 2017, he was honored as a Meritorious Official by the National Wrestling Hall of Fame.

In administrative roles, Hagerty founded the Inter-Collegiate Wrestling Officials Association in 2015 and continues to serve as its Executive Director. He also contributes to USA Wrestling as a coach and was part of the coaching staff for the Olympic training camps in 2012 and 2016. His dedication to developing the sport has been recognized with multiple accolades, including USA Wrestling Developmental Coach of the Year.

Outside the wrestling arena, Hagerty is committed to philanthropy. He directs WrestlingMS, a nonprofit organization dedicated to improving the lives of individuals living with multiple sclerosis by donating bikes and bike packages. An avid cyclist, he balances his professional endeavors with family life, cherishing his roles as a husband, father of four, and grandfather to seven granddaughters.

Connect with Mike at hagshealth.net.

www.ingramcontent.com/pod-product-compliance
Lightning Source LLC
Chambersburg PA
CBHW020547030426
42337CB00013B/994